HEALING THE INFERTILE FAMILY

Strengthening Your Relationship in the Search for Parenthood

HEALING THE INFERTILE FAMILY

Strengthening Your Relationship in the Search for Parenthood

GAY BECKER

UNIVERSITY OF CALIFORNIA PRESS
Berkeley · Los Angeles · London

University of California Press
Berkeley and Los Angeles, California
University of California Press, Ltd.
London, England

First California Paperback Printing 1997

Library of Congress Cataloging-in-Publication Data

Becker, Gaylene.
Healing the infertile family : strengthening your relationship in the search for parenthood / Gay Becker.
p. cm.
Originally published : New York : Bantam Books, © 1990.
Includes bibliographical references and index.
ISBN 0-520-21180-4
1. Marriage. 2. Childlessness. 3. Infertility—Psychological aspects. I. Title.
HQ734.B475 1997
306.87—dc21 97-8565
CIP

0 9 8 7 6 5 4 3 2 1

For Kris, and for Roger

Acknowledgments

Many persons have contributed to the progress of this book. First and foremost, my wholehearted thanks go to those men and women who gave so freely of their time, who willingly relived old pain and examined new ideas so that I might learn something that would benefit others. Although I have changed all names and identifying characteristics of the families who participated, they know who they are. I am deeply grateful for their valuable contributions.

This book is based on research funded by the Academic Senate of the University of California, San Francisco, and by the National Institute on Aging, National Institutes of Health, "Gender and the Disruption of Life Course Structure," RO1 AG08973. This support was essential to the conduct of the research.

Without a doubt, my personal experience, as well as the research itself, has influenced the nature and direction of this book. My friendship with Kristine Grimes Bertelsen has been especially important. It is an uncommon experience for two friends to simultaneously undergo an unexpected life experience, such as infertility, together. Yet that is what happened to Kris and me. We have spent much of our long friendship exploring our identities and lives as women. This included, initially, our fertility and its ramifications for our lives. Later on, our infertility was superimposed on the larger issue. Her willingness to look unflinchingly at every aspect of this experience with me has contributed greatly to the insights I have had about the way women experience this entire phase of life.

Lynda Schmidt has also played a special role, significantly influencing my thinking on issues related to women, men, and relationships. She has been a source of continual inspiration in my own personal odyssey of self-discovery that has taken place as this book unfolded, as well as in my work.

Many thanks to Robert Nachtigall, my research partner in studying infertility, who has contributed greatly to my understanding of infertility and its medical treatment. I am also grateful to the research staff who contributed so much to these projects:

Edwina M. Newsom, project manager; Gary Cook, Jeff Harmon, Seline Szkupinski Quiroga, and Diane Tober, who conducted interviews; Lin Bentley, LaSonya Chatman, Susan Churka-Hyde, Leilani Cuizon-Canalita, Claire Cumings, and Norton Twite, who were involved in various aspects of interview transcription and manuscript production.

Two of my research partners, Sharon Kaufman and Robert Newcomer, have given me ongoing support. Not only did they carry on with our other research endeavors when I was preoccupied, they reviewed papers and proposals and gave me astute comments and suggestions. Robert Newcomer also made the resources of the Institute for Health and Aging, at the University of California, San Francisco, available to me. Without these resources, this book could not have been completed.

Many others have provided all kinds of encouragement in the fifteen years since I began this research. I would especially like to thank Robert Glass, Carl Levinson, Mary Martin, Gay Nadler, Lucile Newman, Marcia Ory, Carolyn Weiner, and Jane Sprague Zones. Lita Teran-Cummings helped to recruit volunteers for the research. I also wish to acknowledge and thank the organizations that helped to recruit participants for the second study: Catholic Charities Adoption Services, Northern California Resolve, and PACT—An Adoption Alliance.

It has been a pleasure to work on this book with Charlene Woodcock at the University of California Press.

I might have abandoned this project long ago had it not been for the enthusiastic support I have received from my friends, from experts in the field of infertility, and from my fellow social scientists. I am very grateful to all of them.

Finally, I would like to thank my husband, Roger Van Craeynest, who has gamely gone through these years of our lives with me. His willingness to tackle our infertility and its effects on our relationship, his tolerance when I made our private life a public matter, and his many anthropological insights about the cultural context in which men and women live out their lives have not only enriched the book, they have kept our relationship lively.

Table of Contents

Foreword

Infertility has no symptoms, it causes no disability, it is invisible. Infertility is not feared except by those who suffer from it, yet with few exceptions, no human experience is as threatening. Whether expressed as a melancholic wistfulness or as a life-consuming rage, its effects on the human psyche—anger, guilt, sadness, isolation, loneliness, frustration, and remorse—are universal. Although infertility is medically unique in that the "patient" is two people, it is particularly unfortunate that men and women experience it in different and often dissonant ways.

Dr. Becker's research over the last two decades is both remarkable and invaluable because it has focused on three critical elements rarely addressed in the scientific infertility literature. The first is the recognition that the "Infertility Epidemic" is a cultural, not biological phenomenon. The second is that infertility's unique effects on peoples' lives are both culturally informed and dominated by gender differences. The third is that the "medicalization" of infertility as witnessed by the extreme technological orientation of modern treatment is itself a major and stressful component of the infertility experience. In this updated edition, Dr. Becker tackles all of these issues.

Couples who have never experienced infertility rarely question the basic cultural expectations of marriage and family building. Infertility, an unwelcome and "unscheduled life transition," forces an often painful conscious examination of this cultural imperative. The unspoken differences in expectations that men and women bring to marriage and childbearing are exacerbated and exaggerated by the experience of infertility. This discrepancy invites polarization. For most women, even those who had willingly and willfully postponed pregnancy, the anxious pall of infertility appears with devastating speed if pregnancy, once intended, is not quickly achieved. Ignoring past career or educational choices or success, women quickly conclude that their very purpose in life is threatened. Although a man may abstractly long for the comfort of roots, marriage, and a stable household, the need to nurture a child is not an urgent aspect of his hormonal or cultural makeup. Men's biological clocks are silent. Beyond an occasional thought about contraception, many men give little, if any, thought to pregnancy and enter adulthood without much anticipation of fatherhood. But for most women, having children is not a hidden agenda, it *is* the agenda.

As a woman becomes preoccupied by the infertility, her husband resents the fact that his partner has become obsessed by this event in their lives and may emotionally withdraw from the turmoil. Disappointed and angry, she questions his commitment to her and his desire for a child. The husband may lament the lack of children, but mostly, he wonders what has happened to his wife. His helplessness and frustration mount as he begins to realize that nothing he says will ease the emotional pain that his partner is experiencing. For both parties, the result is a sense of loneliness and isolation as they suffer through separate struggles.

Healing the Infertile Family is an invaluable tool for patients, physicians, mental health professionals, social scientists, or anyone seeking understanding and insight into the experience of infertility. With a new Introduction that reports on subsequent research, Dr. Becker draws on extensive research-based personal interviews, including new case studies of advanced reproductive technologies. She brings a scholarly but compassionate tone to a skillful exploration of the psychological and cultural meaning of infertility. The medical outcome of infertility treatment is still maddeningly unpredictable, but as a patient of mine told me, "You can't point to infertility as doing either all positive or all negative things. In any relationship that is healthy, things change. That's the way it's been for us with infertility. In the four years now that we've been at it, infertility has done a lot of different things to us. Sometimes it created real barriers between us. Sometimes it's made us feel much closer. It's funny that way, because it seems to shift. But what it has done is made us respect our own strength. We've been going through something terrible, but we've been going through it. We haven't killed each other and we haven't gotten divorced. It's hard to believe sometimes, but I think we're going to be all right, no matter what happens." Perhaps the greatest contribution of *Healing the Infertile Family* is that it is truly about healing.

Robert D. Nachtigall, M.D.
San Francisco
April, 1997

Preface

Infertility is hard to talk about. I know that as a medical anthropologist who has personally experienced fertility problems. I decided to study the issues that surround fertility in mid-life after my own struggle with infertility subsided. I had spent much of the preceding five years trying to navigate a swamp of emotions that encompassed my fertility, my relationship, and the meaning of my life.

During that time I tried *not* to offer myself pat social science answers to the issues that engulfed me. I purposely read nothing because the lure of thinking rather than feeling my way through this unexpected crisis—being businesslike about the whole process—was so appealing. I realized it was a way to *not* deal with the issues. But, as a result, I couldn't invoke the distance my training as a social scientist had given me, a distance that leads ultimately to insight.

What if we *didn't* have children? I had gone blithely through the years not being concerned, not thinking about it, then suddenly it was an issue—not just in my life but in the lives of my friends. An entire year of my life is marked by brown bag lunches on a sunny bench by the bay with a friend, as we escaped our jobs to compare notes on our "progress"—toward decisions, toward our partners' agreement. And then taking the leap—trying to conceive. Life was hopeful and exciting.

Another year is marked by the gray concrete building I next worked in, and the fog of San Francisco that perennially envelops it. Feeling gray inside, I waited for the pregnancy that would take me away from my daily routine and into the next stage of life.

That year I worked side by side with another friend who was struggling with the same issues, only I didn't know it. So private was our pain that we talked about everything *but* our fertility. Years later, when I "came out of the closet," she revealed that—for all the strategies we had developed for dealing with various issues, like the health problems of our aging family members—the *real* issue was something else.

This was just the beginning, *before* Roger and I came up against the big issues, the ones that affected the nuts and bolts of our relationship, that affected our joint and individual concerns, not only about mid-life but about the rest of our lives as well. The ones that can't be articulated in a sentence, or even in a chapter. Much more was to come in the several years that followed, before this story drew to a close.

Once my personal experience was behind me, as I sorted through it and prepared to put it to rest, I realized there was one important ingredient that had helped me to make sense of the whole experience all along—my perspective as an anthropologist. I began to see more clearly that what I knew about individual development over the course of life, about family dynamics, and about the role of culture in our lives had profoundly affected me and my subsequent resolution of the problem. It helped, too, that I was used to working in hospitals and with health professionals, and had spent considerable time analyzing the health care system and its interaction with people's lives. In seeking medical treatment I had been on familiar ground.

When I came out on the other side of this experience and started enjoying life again, I wanted to share what I had learned with others undergoing the same experience. I wanted to make sense out of some of the broader issues that continued to perplex me. I realized there were some missing pieces and hoped that a research project would help to identify what they were.

I believe that knowledge is power, that it gives people autonomy and control over their lives. Understanding ourselves and what is happening to us reduces the sense of powerlessness we feel. It enables us to sort out what we have the power to change from those social and cultural forces that are outside our scope as individuals to alter. I am convinced that understanding, combined with support from others, gives us the tools for insight into ourselves and the situations we find ourselves in, and enables us to transcend whatever befalls us in life.

It's for reasons like this that I have written this book. Sometimes solace is three feet away, like my friend at the next desk, and yet remains invisible because we are caught inexorably in the grip of our own drama. This kind of tunnel vision prevents us from effectively using the resources at our disposal in the short-term. Ultimately, it may prevent us from using our personal experience, however painful, to grow.

This is a time of life when we need both support and insight. Fertility issues create feelings of social isolation. Issues of mid-life may create the same sense of being stranded, alone. Much of the struggle goes on internally, as we ask ourselves endless questions about what we want from life and confront our deepest selves.

Although social scientists strive for objectivity, the issues that interest them most are usually linked in some way with their own personal life experience, no matter how far removed the subject may *appear* to be. And it is usually these issues about which they have the greatest insight. Just as there is an "art" as well as a "science" to medicine, there is a subjective as well as an objective side to social research. On the subjective side is the search for answers that reflect the needs of an inner detective, answers that will somehow help to make better sense of the social scientist's own personal world.

My lifelong search to understand my own kaleidoscope of concerns has led me, throughout my career, to ask questions about how unanticipated change alters the course of life. Anything unexpected alters our route, closing some doors and opening others. In the process, these changes give us life possibilities without end, an exciting—albeit often frightening—way of viewing our own life, since the future is unknowable. My primary aim in following this line of inquiry had been to learn how people create their own continuity *despite* the discontinuous strands that, in actuality, form part of the warp and woof of our lives. As humans, we do strive for continuity, an ongoing effort that never ceases, and in doing so, we strengthen the fabric of our life.

Fertility issues at mid-life fit naturally into this emphasis.

In developing the research, I anticipated that those who could bring themselves to talk about this time in their life would speak with an eloquence born from this intense life experience. I had already noticed many common themes in talking with consumers and professionals in clinical settings and in personal encounters. In carrying out the research, I expected that people's stories of their own lives would reveal new insights into how women and men experience their fertility and their relationship with their partner. What I learned far exceeded my expectations.

Interviews often began with one or both partners commenting that they could not have talked with me six months ago, or a year, or two years earlier. Some said that discussing these issues with me at that time would have been too painful, while others confessed their fear that it would have been too hard on their relationship. Many people did participate only because they shared my conviction that something had to be done to make this entire experience better understood.

As the initial interview began, one or both partners often hung back, afraid of issues emerging that might in some way damage their relationship with each other. Caught by their own compelling stories and the enormity of their feelings, however, women and men forgot their initial hesitation in a few minutes and became engrossed by their own stories. Several hours later, as the interview drew to a close, they often commented that it was a relief to talk about it.

An anthropologist always searches for the hidden key that will unlock the topic and make sense of a vast array of cultural issues. The research project yielded many results and new ideas for future work. Most important, it uncovered the missing link.

In the case of fertility and its problems, the missing link is gender.

Introduction

It has been almost ten years since I wrote *Healing the Infertile Family* but the observations I made then about the effects of infertility on relationships between women and men have been reinforced by subsequent research that I discuss in this updated edition. Shortly after *Healing the Infertile Family* was finished, my research partner, Robert Nachtigall, and I began a much larger study funded by the National Institute on Aging, National Institutes of Health, the goal of which was to pursue further the basic questions we had originally asked about how women and men live with infertility. We undertook a study with 134 couples and 9 women without their partners who were either undergoing medical treatment at the time of the first interview or had completed medical treatment during the preceding three years. People were interviewed several times over a two-year period, enabling us to look more closely at the effects of infertility on women's and men's lives and their relationships with each other over the long term.

We wanted to know several specific things in this second study. First, we wanted to know whether differences we had found in women's and men's response to infertility that I address in this book prevailed in a study with a much larger number of people. Second, we wanted to understand more about how this experience disrupted people's lives and what people did to mediate disruption. Third, we wanted to know how the introduction of advanced reproductive technologies affected people's experience of infertility and in what ways. Although I have subsequently written another book that addresses how people deal with unexpected crises in life[1], *Healing the Infertile Family* continues to be the only book

I have written that examines gender relations and the effects of infertility on couples. In this updated edition, I incorporate new information from the subsequent study, and add case examples of the effects of advanced reproductive technologies such as in vitro fertilization on couples' relationships.

In a pronatalist society such as the United States there is still little room for variation from social norms about parenthood. Inability to biologically reproduce represents a failure to meet cultural norms and affects both men and women.[2] Cultural traditions based on the idea of generation are disrupted. The failure to have children may even be considered to be deviant.[3] The social pressure women and men experience to conceive magnifies the pain of infertility.

My basic goal has been to illustrate how the experience of unwanted childlessness is shaped by cultural meanings—of parenthood, womanhood, and manhood—so that people undergoing infertility can gain an understanding of why they find this experience so difficult. Because of my own experience with infertility, I set out to write a book that would provide practical suggestions for how to deal with the untenable situations in which couples struggling with infertility find themselves. The purpose of this ethnography—the term anthropologists use to refer to the study of a particular topic—is to provide a general readership with a cultural framework for understanding the problem of infertility. This book is an example of what I call "popular ethnography." In the Epilogue I discuss the implications of writing anthropology for the general public.

When I wrote *Healing the Infertile Family,* a set of anthropological ideas guided my thinking, ideas that have continued to develop in the intervening years. These ideas were either in the form of notes following the text or were left out completely. Although readers may still find detailed information in the Notes to various chapters, in the pages that follow I highlight what those ideas are and how they form a framework for thinking about infertility. My discussion of these ideas is entwined with findings from the subsequent research project.

THE SOCIAL AND CULTURAL CONTEXT OF FERTILITY

What drives the unrelenting effort to conceive a child? Why do women and men experience so much anguish when their efforts to conceive are unsuccessful? To answer these questions we need to listen to people's stories and to look beyond them, as well, to identify broad social and cultural forces that affect people's lives. Cultural expectations about the course life will take is one of these forces. The course of life is a cultural phenomenon. That is, in every society women and men have expectations for the course their life will take. These expectations differ somewhat from one culture to another, based on what is considered normal in that culture. People's plans and goals evolve out of these cultural norms for the content and timing of the life course. For example, in many parts of the world people marry and have children at much younger ages than do people in the United States. The anticipated course of life can be seen as a powerful collective image that we share.[4]

Cultural ideas about the course of life as orderly, predictable, and continuous are specific to Western societies, in particular to the United States.[5] Those ideas dictate cultural expectations about marriage and children. Not only do images of the cultural life course dictate people's overall plan for their lives, these images are specific according to gender, ethnic group, and age. Most women, for example, view the family life cycle as occurring in an orderly, continuous way and view themselves as having responsibility for maintaining the continuity of the family. Children symbolize continuity between the past and the future. When children are expected but conception does not occur, the anticipated course of life is disrupted.

When women and men are immersed in infertility treatment, it is hard to keep in mind that infertility is primarily a social problem, not a medical problem. It is only recently that this social condition has been recast as a disease.[6] The social science literature of the 1960s and 1970s addressed the problem of "involuntary childlessness," a social condition defined by the unwanted absence of children. As this social problem assumed greater proportions, largely as a consequence of delayed childbearing, medical treatment was increasingly sought.[7] This shift has occurred in tandem with increased medical emphasis on infertility, including increasing numbers of physicians who specialize in reproductive endocrinology, an escalation of research on infertility, and the development of new reproductive technologies. This shift in perspective, from viewing unwanted childlessness as a social problem to a medical problem, reflects a redefinition of health as well as increasing domination of health-related concerns by biomedicine.

The process of identifying a problem as health-related and turning to medical treatment to conceive a child is called medicalization.[8] Why has childlessness become medicalized? The value of children and their pivotal place in the social organization of society appears to be central to the medicalization of childlessness.[9] Although Snowden found that the ability to procreate is a cultural expectation for men,[10] cultural expectations for women's social roles are shaped more broadly by their child-bearing capacity. Women take responsibility for the family life cycle and become the instrumental partner in pursuing plans to parent. Their sense of responsibility for bearing children is an active ingredient in the pursuit of medical treatment for infertility.[11]

Although infertility is not a disease, it is treated like one in the health care system. The way in which infertility is medically defined and treated is based on biomedical assumptions that lead to the categorization of infertility as a disease entity, a medical statement that it is abnormal to be unable to reproduce biologically. Medical evaluation for infertility identifies physical "defects" through the identification of one or more infertility factors. These bodily differences from a medically delineated norm are identified in the presence of apparent good health.[12]

CHANGING EFFECTS OF MEDICAL TREATMENT

Since this book first appeared, new reproductive technologies have begun to make a significant impact on traditional notions about conception and parenthood in United States society. New technologies are challenging old ideas about conception. For example, fertilization of an ovum may take place in a petri dish rather than inside a woman's body. Some children are born who have the same genetic material as their parents while others do not.

But at the same time that they are fostering innovation, those technologies are reinforcing traditional ideas about the primacy of parenthood through biology by creating an endless array of medical treatments designed to produce a biological child. Thirty years ago anthropologist David Schneider published a book, *American Kinship,* that questioned popular conceptions of kinship. He suggested that, although people in the U.S. view kinship as a *natural* system, kinship is a *symbolic* system.[13] That is, the way Americans think about kinship is not the only way that kinship is viewed around the world. Indeed, very few societies think of kinship as people do in the United States, where kinship is based either on blood ties or on ties by marriage. Of the two types of ties, blood ties are seen as more binding than ties of marriage. In contrast, many societies are organized into clans, which may be extremely large, and everyone in the clan is considered to be a relative. In such societies the web of family relationships is likely to be much more extensive, with different sorts of implications for people who experience infertility.

What the American kinship system means for women and men experiencing infertility, in practical terms, is that people who choose to gain validation for other forms of kinship, such as adoption, face a struggle because adoption is not part of the United States system of kinship.[14] Because it is not seen as natural, adoption is often viewed as second-best. People must work to fit it into a reconfigured view of the family. Doing so entails a willingness to depart from traditional notions about what a family is and means that, in order to entertain an alternative approach to family creation, people must significantly change how they think about the meaning of family. Advanced reproductive technologies, even while they are expanding the meaning of family, constrain those meanings by underscoring the importance of biology.

We have found in both studies that the majority of men favor adoption, while the majority of women do not—at least not until they have tried every medical means of bringing about a conception. Adoption is seldom women's first choice for several reasons: they have become invested in medical treatment, they want to experience pregnancy and childbirth, and they want a biological child. They may want to persist with advanced reproductive technologies before turning to adoption.

In the research that was undertaken after this book was completed, we found some distinct changes to have taken place in the experience of infertility. The length of time that couples stay in medical treatment and the amount of money they spend on treatment has greatly escalated since our first study. As new medical therapies become available, couples often feel compelled to try those therapies before they can bring closure to medical treatment.[15] The majority of those who are not successful in conceiving during medical treatment turn only as a last resort to other options such as adoption, fostering children, or remaining childless. At this point, their emotional and financial reserves may be completely depleted, and the work of resolving infertility may be harder to address because they have given so much energy to medical treatment.

How does this extended effort to conceive a biological child affect a couple's relationship?[16] To answer that question we must take a closer look at the role of gender, not simply at the role of infertility. The vast majority of work by social scientists in the past two decades affirms the social and cultural basis of gender definitions. That is, just as kinship is not rooted in a universal set of facts, neither is gender. Meanings of "male" and "female" reflect culturally-imposed differences that are based in the structures of a society; they are not just about natural differences.[17] Gender constitutes a basic dimension of social organization, and encompasses socially constructed relationships, cultural meanings, and identities through which biological sex becomes socially significant.[18] One way that gender is institutionalized is through families. Definitions of what constitutes a family have altered and expanded radically in recent times, further challenging traditional notions of family.[19] Despite such changes, traditional notions about gender and family prevail. In this book we will examine people's efforts to live up to traditional notions of gender and gender roles in the United States, explore how they struggle with dominant ideas about gender that they are unable to live out, and trace different ways in which they seek to resolve this challenge.

In *Healing the Infertile Family* I talk about culturally-imposed differences between women and men and especially about efforts to reconcile those differences. But it is also possible to see culturally-imposed differences in responses between persons of the same gender. Those differences reflect their fertility status and are based on gender-specific cultural assumptions about fertility. In the body of the book I discuss differences in response between men who are diagnosed as being infertile and men whose fertility is not questioned. Both studies uncovered some specific differences. Men who are diagnosed as having male factor infertility have a more negative emotional response to infertility than men who do not have an infertility factor in three respects: feelings of stigma, sense of loss, and diminished self-esteem. This difference reflects men's response to cultural expectations about fertility: infertile men are reacting to cultural attitudes about male infertility, which profoundly affect their sense of self, even if their infertility remains hidden from others. But all men report a sense of role failure regardless of whether or not they are diagnosed as infertile. (Role failure is the inability to meet cultural expectations for one's roles as an adult, such as marital partner.) In other words, regardless of their fertility status, men are deeply distressed by conflicts they experience in their relationships with their partners and by their inability to solve the problem of infertility quickly.[20]

This response to infertility on the part of men reflects cultural expectations about the male role in the United States apart from specific cultural expectations about fertility.

In contrast, no differences were found among women in their emotional response to infertility regardless of whether or not a female infertility factor is found. All women report a sense of stigma, perceptions of loss, role failure, and loss of self esteem. That is, it doesn't matter if a woman is diagnosed as infertile or not, her response is the same as other women undergoing infertility treatment. This finding tells us something about United States cultural expectations about fertility, that women view their fertility more globally than do men, and that their sense of responsibility for biological reproduction is all-encompassing and is not simply linked to a physical diagnosis of fertile or infertile.

In *Healing the Infertile Family,* I focus on conflicts that women and men experience in the first few years of the discovery of infertility and its treatment and their efforts to resolve both their conflicts with each other and over infertility. Although such conflicts are experienced by couples as being interpersonal, these conflicts have their roots in gender-specific cultural expectations. But what happens in the long term? In the second study people were interviewed in every stage of this experience, several times over a much longer period of time. This included couples who had recently discovered their infertility and had been in medical treatment for a year or less; couples who were in the midst of basic infertility treatment; couples who were undergoing advanced reproductive technologies or had abandoned efforts to conceive and were considering adoption or childlessness; and couples who felt they had brought a close to their infertility and resolved it, either because they had successfully conceived or adopted, or because they were reconciled to life without children. Thus, we were able to observe couples undergoing transitions from one phase of infertility to another.

With this wealth of new information from over two hundred people, it now seems safe to say that infertility does not destroy relationships, at least not in the vast majority of cases. Couples are often able to refocus by recognizing the impact of culturally-derived gender expectations on their relationship. Once couples get a grip on the overall problem of infertility and work out strategies for how to deal with it, they persevere. Those strategies are outlined in this book based on my observations in the initial study. In the second study I was able to observe how people develop and use these strategies successfully over long periods of time.

This is not to say that ongoing tensions or specific pressure points do not exist, because they do. But if partners are able to relate to the other person's perspective and if, as a couple, they can develop ways to support each other, their relationship can thrive and mature from this experience. The great majority of couples in the second study—those who had been undergoing infertility for three years or more—with few exceptions, ended up together rather than apart on the issue of infertility. They had developed the tools they needed to get through this experience together. I outline those tools in this book.

What are the ongoing tensions in couples' relationships that are caused by infertility? One experienced by almost every couple: infertility treatment is women's work. Because of the way infertility treatment is structured, men are less involved, even if it is their infertility that is being addressed in medical treatment. Infertility treatment is still carried out primarily on women, providing a cogent example of how gender expectations are embedded in social institutions, such as the delivery of health care. Over the long term women may get tired of being the more responsible party and resent their partners being less involved. Women's preoccupation with medical treatment is a related tension. Men may deeply resent this. There are ways of ameliorating these problems. I discuss them in the pages that follow.[21]

Like other medical frontiers that offer new technologies, infertility treatment gives couples hope. Treatment often does result in a conception taking place. Nevertheless, this process is not without its costs—costs that go far beyond the financial expense of pursuing infertility treatment. These other costs are hard to calculate but they contribute significantly to the conflict women and men may experience in undergoing infertility treatment. They include loss of self-esteem, a reduced sense of autonomy, loss of bodily knowledge, altered self-image, loss of a sense of control, and a sense of difference from others.

In both studies women and men experienced an assault on the body as infertility treatment got underway. This was because infertility treatment inadvertently reinforced their feelings of failure to live up to gendered cultural expectations about fertility. Because we followed people for so long in the second study, we were able to observe the long-term effects of this assault on the body. When people remained in infertility treatment for years at a time, their identity and their view of their body changed in profound ways. This was especially true for women, as the primary recipients of medical care. Examples of the effects on women and men abound, but perhaps the most dramatic example occurred when women—pregnant at last—were unable to believe they were pregnant, and once they finally grasped the fact, were unable to enjoy their pregnancy because of their fears that the conception would not result in a healthy baby. While it is true that some women's fears were realized, in the majority of cases women experienced uneventful pregnancies.

Further indication that women's identity is changed in the long term is given by our finding from the second study that all women in the post-treatment group reported they continued to think about their infertility, talk to others about infertility, and try to help other women undergoing infertility, even if they had completed their family. Moreover, they reported ongoing effects of infertility on their lives. These issues were usually specific to the particular route they had ultimately taken, such as adoption, the use of a donor, health risks they had taken in undergoing advanced reproductive technologies, or the meaning of living without children.

What are the pressure points couples experience and when do they occur? Most of these pressures are associated with medical treatment. When couples begin to consider advanced reproductive technologies or adoption, the cost of infertility may become an issue as never before. Advanced reproductive technologies necessitate advance planning, and couples start to talk about making major outlays of income from savings accounts and other resources. Or, as is increasingly the case, they may begin talking about borrowing money to offset medical or adoption costs. Neither advanced reproductive technologies or adoption is a sure thing, although adoption appears to have a higher likelihood of eventual success. Men often feel their primary contribution to the joint effort of dealing with infertility, apart from emotional support, is to be responsible for handling the money to finance infertility treatment. Men may be especially daunted by the cost of these procedures. What is more, men may be more concerned about the medical risks their partner may be taking than their partner is.[22]

The question of ending medical treatment, which may or may not be part of the decision-making process around advanced reproductive technologies, is another pressure point. What happens when one partner wants a child no matter what and the other partner doesn't? What happens when one partner wants to adopt and the other partner doesn't? Sometimes women and men negotiate over infertility at an earlier stage of treatment and only later do complexities arise. A common scenario from the second study was this: he agrees to support her pursuit of a biological child in exchange for her support for a career change he plans to make after they conceive. But if the effort to conceive seems to be endless and eats up all their financial resources while he continues to postpone the changes he wants to initiate, conflict inevitably ensues. Sometimes this scenario is complicated by practical issues, such as being unable to quit a job because work-related insurance pays for infertility treatment. It is times like these when women and men most need the tools they have developed for living through infertility together.

The findings from this research suggest that it is extremely important to try to maintain a sense of balance about the possibilities. Infertility treatment often helps people solve the problem of childlessness. But keep in mind that solutions to infertility are often complex. Even when people succeed in keeping a balance, there are bound to be some inroads on identity. Infertility is such a profound disruption to people's expectations about life, it cannot simply be forgotten.

When people experience infertility, they collide with a range of dominant assumptions in society—about kinship, gender, and fertility. In seeking to bring about change in their lives, people must wrestle with those dominant, taken-for-granted ideas which may represent a perspective very different from their own experience as they confront infertility. This struggle may challenge them to search for alternatives that create a better fit with their definitions of themselves. In order to resolve infertility, people need to move beyond cultural assumptions. Doing so takes time and energy. The interim period between the time that people identify a fracture in their plans to parent and the time that they resolve their infertility is a time for people to rethink their assumptions about what life is about and what they want from it. Although it may seem to those living through it as a stagnant time of waiting for something that never seems to happen, it is much more accurate to characterize this time as one of creative ferment, as people attempt to come to terms with life as it is, rather than as it was expected to be.[23]

CHAPTER 1

IDENTITY AND FERTILITY

> It's the ultimate humiliation for a man. It's worse than a lot of things—physical disability, being short. Not being able to reproduce—it's the worst. And Sally thinks it is the worst thing for a woman.*

Jerry sat slumped on the couch, his long legs sprawled out in front of him. He addressed his comment to the floor in front of him in a voice full of pain. Sally sat upright in the other corner of the couch, her legs tucked under her. In an angry voice, she said,

> You said you wanted to know about our infertility? Well, I have a question, too. What I want to know is, 'Why us?' He has no sperm, and my mucus stinks.

Jerry interjected:

> To me, it's cutting off your balls.

Sally turned to him:

> Well, what am I cutting off me when I can't have a baby?

Jerry, taking her hand, said in a shaky voice:

> I know that. I'm just talking.

By now, Sally was crying.

*All names and identifying characteristics have been changed to protect anonymity.

> I don't have balls.

Jerry explained to me,

> For us, infertility is failing. If Sally can't have a baby, she's failing as a woman, and I'm failing as a man.

Reproduction of the species is a basic expectation people hold. Jerry and Sally have planned their lives around this shared cultural assumption, that they are naturally endowed with fertility. This is what evolution is supposed to be about. Jerry and Sally believe their basic purpose as human beings is to reproduce, to perpetuate the species. This is their part in the broader scheme of things, in the enormous tapestry of humankind. That's what culture is based on—people. Each generation of children makes it possible for the culture to continue. Children symbolize the future—the continuity of the family, the march of generations, the renewal of life. Immortality.

This is no small undertaking. When we decide to have children, not only do we live out the path we have chosen through life, we link ourselves to the rest of humanity. The task ahead of us is greater than the sum of our partnership with each other. It is the perpetuation of the species.

As a result of these expectations, faith in our fertility is embedded in our identity from the time we are small. So when fertility is questioned, it is a threat to identity. The most deep-seated ideas men and women hold about their masculinity and femininity are challenged. They have failed to meet their expectations for themselves. The humiliation they feel goes beyond a biological inability to have a child to encompass the meaning of manhood and womanhood.

What it means to be a man or a woman is at the very heart of our identity. We have a strong emotional response to the very words. We identify with them. Words like manly and womanly, masculine and feminine, conjure up a host of images. Images of ourselves. When women and men don't measure up to these images, they begin to wonder who they are.

> I'm not that big, but I feel like a horse around people, and just masculine. No chest, no nothing. I'm not that big, but I feel like a eunuch.
>
> —Marsha

Fertility is not only linked to masculinity and femininity, it stands for productivity, growth, and continuity. *Webster's Dictionary* imparts the full power of the word:

> *Producing abundantly; rich in resources or invention; fruitful; prolific; causing or helping fertility; able to produce young, seeds, fruit, pollen, spores; capable of development into a new individual. Fertile implies a producing or power of producing, fruit or offspring, and may be used figuratively of the mind.*

If there was any question about why fertility triggers such intense feelings, now it's clear. Fertility is culturally loaded. These words are alive with meaning—a blueprint for success. If men and women don't meet these expectations to become parents, they channel their sense of failure through their gender identity.

Down through the ages, this mission has been so ingrained in each of us—this cultural and biological ethic to reproduce—that it has never been questioned. Until recently.

Change began with the revolution in technology that gave us the Pill. And with the Pill came a revolution in our thinking. Birth control has probably been around as long as people have. But it wasn't very effective. Inadequate birth control shaped attitudes in the other direction—people thought of children as inevitable. And immediate.

But with the arrival of the Pill, attitudes about having children began to change. Especially ideas about when to start. Suddenly, there were choices about the future. As a result, many of us postponed childbearing while we explored the rest of our universe. As our identity developed—as we began to discover who we are and proclaim it through our actions and ideas—we did as we pleased, whether it was to get an education, sail around the world, or start a career.

And we met the partner who has given so much meaning to our life. We went on together, sometimes for years, savoring the life we created together. Until one day we found ourselves in a bind. What to do next?

> We've been going together and known each other almost three years, and I'd say after the first year we talked it over. But then we just went on. But last year, because of my age, I made it very clear that if he was interested in our relationship continuing, then let's have a child. Because I was so late—so old—that every minute counted.
>
> —Sandra

As this journey begins, we may be daunted by the immensity of this undertaking. The changes a child will bring, the unknown future it will help to create, seem formidable—sometimes overwhelming. The idea of being one tiny cog in the wheel of life adds to the enormity of the undertaking. Its meaning for each of us—as a woman, as a man, and for our relationship—is profound.

In this book I talk about what happens once the decision to have children is made, especially if it doesn't happen exactly the way it is planned. The whole scenario about whether or not to have a baby, and when to have one, may get pretty complicated. Because when the script was changed, we lost sight of two important details.

The first is biology. There's the question of how long a woman is fertile. How long can she wait? Fertility in women starts to decline after the age of 30. And the longer women wait, the fewer children they have.

What about men? Not much is known about male fertility. It has not received much scientific attention until recently. So far, we are assuming that men's fertility goes on undiminished. But we don't know that much about fertility in men yet, so it's hard to say.

The second is culture. Men and women are different—sometimes. One of those times is when we face the prospect of parenthood. We're not ready at the same time, we don't have the same agenda. We weren't raised to think the same way about having children, or about what family means. Not only that, no matter how much feminism has been at work in the last twenty years, when we were small, boys were raised to work and girls were raised to have babies.

The way we are raised leaves its imprint. Culture is a strong force in our lives. It is played out in our parents' expectations for us and in the locker room at school. It pervades those cliques of giggling girls and rowdy boys, of which we once were part. It is lived out in many microscopic ways, from the food we eat to the clothes we wear, from the way we talk to babies to the way we answer the traffic cop giving us a ticket. Our culture gives us rules for behavior and ways of thinking about things. It shapes the way we see the world and how we get along in daily life. It dictates what we do and how we think, sometimes in spite of ourselves. Along with biology, culture is why men and women are different from each other. And why fertility becomes so charged when we are ready to proceed with having children.

So when a couple starts talking about having children, harmony may go out the window, along with a lot of assumptions they share about how much they are alike. And how easy it is to get along. And how smoothly their lives will unfold. So intimately known to each other five years ago, and even last month, they may suddenly feel like strangers. During dinners out and weekends by the sea, she brings up babies and he brings up freedom. What is happening to their intimacy? To their relationship? Is this just the beginning? How can they keep what they have and still move on to the next step in life?

This book explores what happens between women and men as they start down this road. It examines what happens when things don't go according to plan. And it makes suggestions for what to do about it—how to successfully navigate the issues and avoid the pitfalls at this stage of life.

Most of the talking is done by about forty people—twenty couples who have gone through this turning point in their lives and emerged strong and resilient as they turn to the next stage of life. They recount experiences I have heard repeatedly in the research I conducted for this book.* They reflect on new insights and old pain. They are the voices of experience, as they describe changes—both subtle and profound—they have undergone. They are voices of wisdom, a wisdom that all of us with similar experiences can find in ourselves. What are the paths that lead to solutions? That lead to new self-discovery? That strengthen our relationship? That lead us to peace and resolution? In this book I give you some answers to these questions, and offer some guidelines that I hope will enable you to deal effectively with your infertility and your relationship.

THE MEANING OF FAMILY

What does it mean to be a family? Do we all share the same set of assumptions about the meaning of the word? Who are we talking about? It sounds straightforward, but it's not. Because men and women often have different ideas about what the word *family* means.

Sandra and Tony, as they reached a crossroads in their relationship, found out just how complicated these differences can be.

> SANDRA: I feel very strongly that having children—family—is one of the highest priorities in my life. So I have had a lot of intense feelings about it—that family is basically the most important thing—and children, the next generation, the future.

Tony, her partner, viewed the future differently:

> We're not married yet, although we've been trying to get

*See Epilogue for a description of the research project.

> pregnant. I would argue that the fact we are sharing our lives and our economies and we sleep together, we live together, we eat together, says that essentially we are just the same as being married, that we are a family. But it's not, in Sandra's mind. To her, being unmarried is not being whole.

We usually share the expectation that we will have our own family. But the so-important details of how this will happen may differ considerably in our minds. Like Sandra, women usually think of children as the expression of family. But men may not. Like Tony, men usually see the partnership as the epitome of family. They feel complete. Women tend to look at their partnership in a broader framework—the family life cycle.

Jenny and Matt, looking back over their relationship, marvel at how blind they were to these differences when they married:

> MATT: I was getting married for companionship. I was not getting married for kids. I was mainly thinking about her, and that children would be something natural that would come along eventually. Children weren't something I was opposed to, not something I was frightened of. But I was naive when it came to being married—about what relationships mean, and just growing with a person, and change. So children were going to be part of this later on. I didn't think about it.

> JENNY: I was real purposeful, on the other hand, I was plotting. I got married because I wanted to have kids. I really was not into being married, ever. I really had no need for getting married. But we moved back here, and his family is here, and they put pressure on us.
>
> So I got married because I thought, 'Well, it's time. If I'm going to have kids, I better do it now.'

How does this happen? A couple spends so much time together as their relationship develops, talking and dreaming, sharing their past lives and their hopes for the future. It seems unlikely, but it's not. Jenny and Matt are not unique. They are typical.

Couples make assumptions about each other, that he thinks like she does, that they are alike. They second-guess each other, they read each other's mind. This positive identification with each other—this feeling of being almost one—propels them into the relationship.

Once the relationship has formed, perspective is lost. It's hard—nearly impossible—to see each other clearly anymore. This isn't a problem in itself—it's how relationships evolve. But the myopia both partners develop as the relationship grows blinds them to their differences as a man and a woman.

Our culture camouflages these differences. This is the age of androgyny. Sometimes partners dress the same as each other, sometimes they look the same. They often share the same ideas. Besides, they are supposed to be a team. A modern team. Men change diapers and women take out the garbage. Roles get reversed. Sometimes men stay home with the kids, while women go to work. Isn't that so?

Well, not very often. It may be a great idea but its time hasn't come, apparently.

> You know, women bear kids and men develop hobbies. I have so many hobbies I could accept a childless alternative. But Laura couldn't.
>
> —Stan

As men and women recognize their differences, they try to untangle the suddenly snarled knot in the relationship. Belinda and Al sort through a host of differences—in their gender, in their families, and in their expectations—in search of answers:

> AL: Even though there's a child waiting in the wings for us eventually—even though I will love the kid—there is still a primary thing of Belinda needing to have a child, and so it's going to happen. It's not, 'Me first.' I think I could go through the rest of life without a child. I would be a little sad that that was the case, but with the things I do now—the

activities I am involved in—my lifestyle makes a child an imposition. It definitely would be—it would require changes that I would be willing to make when it is necessary. But I don't look forward to making them. I guess at least I'm being straightforward.

BELINDA: I knew you felt that way. I wondered if you were going to say it.

AL: You mean, be willing to be conscious of it?

BELINDA: Yes. I wish there were a different way. I wish having a child would be as important to you but it's not. You would be okay if we didn't have children. But I can't imagine not having a child in the family. There were five kids in my family when I was growing up. That was what you do, if you're a woman. I want the feeling of being needed and nurturing. That's what I need to do.

AL: In my family there were four of us. The only one who was really into the family scene was my mother. My father was inwardly directed, like I am, and my sister ended up that way. In my childhood the typical evening after dinner was everyone went in their separate directions pretty much and were self-entertained.

BELINDA: Whereas my family is extremely loud and sort of obnoxious. We don't interact emotionally but we interact. And what you have told me about your background is that you didn't interact in your family—at least not on a surface level.

Reflecting on these differences, she concludes:

Maybe men are not necessarily *against* the family, but just not as into having a family. But men go along with it because people have kids—this is what you do.

THE FAMILY LIFE CYCLE

Not everyone grows up to become a parent. Some people choose not to have children, while others delay childbearing and then drift into childlessness because they realize they like their lifestyle just the way it is. But the cultural expectation is that we become parents in adulthood. Parenthood, rather than marriage, stands for full responsibility as an adult.

> I hear so many assumptions from people, like, 'Well, I just don't think you can really grow up until you have children.' And then a variation on that one is, 'You'll never be mature unless you have children because you'll always be so self-centered.' I have seen too many self-centered parents to know that one isn't true.
>
> —Susan

Parenthood is a pivotal stage of the human life cycle. How we think about parenting is central to the way we think about life itself. Because parenthood is the thread that links the generations to each other. Our ability to pass on our experiences in life to younger generations gives meaning to our lives. Erik Erikson calls this "generativity." Nurturing the generations that follow us—the need that Belinda expressed—makes it possible for us to round out our lives. It becomes increasingly important as we go through life. Generativity gives life its form and meaning throughout most of the life cycle. This is how we re-create ourselves, by passing on our storehouses of knowledge—our beliefs, traditions, and ideas—to others.

There are other ways to nurture younger generations—parenthood is *not* the only way! But it is the one we automatically think of.

Not only do we start to get ready for parenthood as children and escalate these activities as we become adults, we look ahead to later life with the idea that our children will grow up and start their own families. And then we will eventually become grandparents, and possibly even great-grandparents, all the time watching the generations unfold.

> I always believed that I would be a father and that I would have a family and grandchildren and the whole bit. I'm the third boy in a family of five. Raising us was a full-time job.
>
> —Russ

> I was very close to my grandmother, and I want that to continue, I mean in cycles. For me not to have a child is the end of that cycle. I really believe that—if I didn't I probably would stop trying to get pregnant.
>
> —Sally

THE UNFOLDING OF GENDER DIFFERENCES

We learn how to become parents by watching our own parents. Expectations about parenthood organize our lives, even in childhood. Little girls, for example, are supposed to play with dolls, learn to sew, and help Mom with the dishes, while little boys play with trains, learn sports, and help Dad with the plumbing. Times have changed, and the gender modeling children undergo has loosened up a lot. But when we were small, behavior that fit with what girls are expected to do, or what boys are expected to do, got applauded. We knew when we picked something that wasn't approved for our gender—we got labeled. As tomboys. Or as sissies.

> I got very intense, very clear, very verbalized feelings from my mother. I come from a family of four, and my mother was more focused on children than on any other adult as long as I can remember. So it was very much an approved and intimate part of growing up.

> I remember when my mother was pregnant with my brother and afterward wanting very much to take care of the baby. And I can even remember the fantasy of him as my baby. I was six when he was born and really playing out that fantasy, being the little mommy and having a baby. Only instead of baby dolls I had my real live brother.
>
> —Sandra

Growing up, women are raised by their mothers to nurture—to become caregivers. Mothers tell their daughters stories of their pregnancies, and how they gave birth. They tell them stories of their own childhood. "When I was five, they put me on a chair so I could reach the stove, and I cooked for the whole family." There is a message in this story. In fact, it's more than a message, it's an expectation. Women are raised to live out these expectations.

> She never gave me any direct messages. She never said a woman's purpose in being born is to procreate. Yet I always felt all those things. And she was a career woman, a very successful one. But she stopped working to raise us. She got a phone call from New York once, offering her a very important job. She turned it down, and I can remember arguing with her. 'Why?' And she said, 'Well, I have to take care of you.' I was probably close to being a teenager and my sister was probably 7 or 8. She didn't really have that much caring to do.
>
> —Laura

The message is clear. Raising children is women's work. According to our mothers, it is our main job in life.

> It harks back to my roots, my origins, that the only reason for getting married is to have children, and certainly the only reason for sex.
>
> —Sandra

What do fathers tell their sons? "When I was your age I had a paper route. Why don't you get one?" What do they say about relationships? "The first time I saw your mother, she was running across an open field, her hair flying. I thought she was the most beautiful girl in the world." There are messages in these stories, too: "Work hard"; "Relationships are romantic."

Do fathers tell their sons anything else? What do mothers tell them? How do men's expectations about children evolve? Men don't talk much about what their fathers—or their mothers—ever said to them about having a family. Men may not think much about having a family, except in general, until it becomes an issue in the relationship.

> I don't know what I wanted. I didn't really want children that much. I just assumed we would have them.
>
> —Jerry

> I've always been an iffy sort of person when it comes to family life. The only constraint that I ever put on it was that if I ever had kids I would have more than one. I was an only child and as I grew up I always said to myself, 'Boy, I never want to live in a family like this.' I used to talk to walls because there wasn't another kid there. And the family life was boring. They were involved with each other, not with me.
>
> —Jeff

> I really didn't have a vision of having children, not at all. There wasn't a goal of being a parent. That wasn't there. I didn't really see myself as married and settled down. I have always been more involved in the here and now—how do I cope with whatever is going on—rather than being a planner.
>
> —Al

Some men do have very strong feelings about having children. And if so, it's usually because the importance of family was spelled out growing up.

> I like my family. I come from a big family, and we have always been very close. I would like to have a family. I don't

> want to raise heifers or horses. I just don't envision never having kids, so even the idea of being childless is a very big change. Maybe I would come around to that but it would be like moving to Zimbabwe. It's just something I have never thought of. It would take a lot to convince me to change my mind.
>
> —Hal

What's the upshot of all these messages? Of this minutiae of everyday life social scientists call socialization? The reverberations are endless. When women and men grow up, we are distinct from each other. Our view of relationships isn't the same. We comprehend the family differently. And we develop a plan for our life that diverges from each other's in subtle ways.

WOMEN'S PURPOSE IN LIFE

Most of us can remember as kids saying, "Dad, can I . . . ?", and the response usually was, "Ask your mother," leaving us with the impression that it's Mom who is responsible for the family. As a result, men and women agree with each other about something important—one thing that keeps us on course as we navigate through these unexpected shoals: Primary responsibility for continuing the family life cycle lies with women.

As we go through life, men and women periodically scan an inner bulletin board of assignments—assignments that change in each stage of life—to make sure we are up to date on our roles. If we see our name up there, we mobilize. If we don't, we relax.

As Stan and Laura describe their expectations growing up, we can hear the difference in how their role expectations formed:

> STAN: I grew up in a small town. It was very family oriented. On vacations we went camping. I was born right after the war [World War II] during the baby boom. There were kids everywhere.

I'm the oldest. I have a sister four years younger than me. It was a really whole growing up. I didn't feel anything was missing. Laura talks about how quiet my parents are, and it's true, they are very quiet, very unemotional. But I never had any sense of it being abnormal or weird or unusual or bad. And that really stays with me because I don't feel anything is missing in me. I feel like they did a good job of raising me. There was love there.

And projecting that growing up out—it's funny. I never said, 'I want to have kids.' But at the same time, I always assumed I would. But I never felt the need for it, unlike Laura. It's like something I'd like to have that I don't feel any immediate need for—I just think, 'Yeah, I'll have one someday.'

LAURA: My desire to be a mother has always been so strong that even as a child I always believed I would never be a mother because I wanted it so badly. Gee, it sounds really gruesome, the truth.

That first gynecologist I went to gave me a chart [a basal body temperature chart] and he said, 'There's nothing wrong with you.' And I kept saying, 'There is, I just know there is.' When I was saying that, I was thinking in my head, 'There has to be because I want this so badly—I'm sure there's something wrong with me.'

STAN: I don't have the intensity about it that Laura has. I could go either way. I think it would be perfectly natural to have children, so I don't have any desire not to have them. But it's not the same driving need that she has. It's just not the same tragedy.

Why is a woman's need for a child so intense as she reaches her thirties? Has she suddenly discovered that something is missing? Yes. It's called her purpose in life, handed down by her mother, by her aunts, by her grandmothers.

> When I'm 50, I would rather say I have children than I don't have children. I would regret not having children. That leaves the potential for too big an emptiness. I'm not about to chance it.
>
> —Doris

No matter how women feel about their purpose as women—whether they accept childbearing as their purpose in life or are ambivalent about it—this idea is a finely spun heritage that cannot be ignored. As women enter their thirties, they have to deal with it—they can't put it off any longer. Because until it is faced, it is not going to be resolved.

> I'm 32, so you know it's critical to make up my mind. I think I've come to the idea that I can live without children. I think I can do that.
>
> I didn't want to have children in my first marriage. That was something I always knew. But when I met Russ things were different; that seemed to be something that we could enjoy together. But it's never been something that I've been yearning for because it would be a biological void if I don't do it or I can't do it.
>
> —Carrie

Whether or not to have children is usually a conscious, ongoing consideration as women reach adulthood. Linked with the other concerns of life, it is never far from center stage. Because someday soon a decision must be made.

> It seems hard to believe now, but when I was in high school I went through a phase where I thought, 'No, I'm never going to have children,' and I was real militant—sort of feminist stuff. I think that had a lot to do with going along with what everybody else was doing and thinking, and exploring options without really thinking about what they would mean in terms of my life.
>
> Then, when I was in my late twenties and we were

> thinking about getting married, I started to get real tempted about having kids. I realized I might not have a real interesting job all my life. You can't just put everything in one place. I thought if I focused completely on my career, I might end up real disappointed. That's when we started to plan.
>
> —Susan

For most women, having children gradually becomes a priority. Even if it is put on the back burner at first. Even if women are not conscious of this wish.

But many women are.

> I have always loved babies. I remember a neighbor had a child, and I would go help her with her baby. I would follow them around. I was about 5. There was never a question about having children someday. This is the most unconflicted thing I have ever done.
>
> —Celia

> I don't know what age I started thinking of this, or if I was even told, but as a kid I became aware of the fact that some women couldn't have children. I thought, 'If a doctor ever told me I could never have children, I would probably kill myself.' I just couldn't think about going through life without them.
>
> —Dorene

> There has never been a time when I thought I would not have children. I still, to this day, can't imagine my life without children.
>
> —Theresa

> For me, I have always wanted a child. Always. And that has never diminished. It has just gotten more so with time.
>
> —Sally

Women, as part of the responsibility they carry for the family life cycle, often make children a requirement in negotiating the relationship. Mothering isn't just a role—it's an identity.

> You are just programmed all your life to think that you are going to have this experience. It is part of your whole being.
>
> —Judy

When Dorene gave Kenny an ultimatum about their relationship, he amended his vision of the future to be compatible with hers, a necessity for their relationship to continue:

> DORENE: One of my conditions of getting married was that we have children. He said that he wasn't sure he wanted to do that, being older, and he didn't know if he wanted to make that kind of commitment. Then he decided that, yeah, that was something he wanted to do. We started trying right away. As soon as we got married, probably even a month or two before we got married, we decided we would go for it.
>
> KENNY: I was somewhat apprehensive about having children. I was married before. I had three stepchildren from that marriage. My ex-wife was not interested in having more children, even when we first got married. The last thing on her mind was having more children. So I just never thought about having children. It never entered my mind.
>
> I think my resistance at the outset with Dorene was the fear of approaching age, of getting older and never doing it before. Then all of a sudden there was the realization that it might happen somehow. I became excited. I wanted kids. So that is when I got to the point of matching Dorene's level of wanting to be a parent. I wasn't forced into it. But I was certainly apprehensive.

Women who feel some ambivalence may be less decisive. Carrie thought she wanted a child but her motivation was lukewarm. Free of a driving purpose, she and Russ negotiated the children issue with flexibility and humor:

> It was an issue that we wanted to discuss before we got really involved to see where we stood on that topic. So many people have different opinions in this day and age, whether they don't want to have children, whether they want to pursue a career, some want to have four kids. So we talked about it and we decided we'd like to have one child and that would be a good round number.

Sometimes women assume that men really want children but they don't know their own minds.

> DORIS: I thought you became enamored with the idea progressively. I don't know how you felt at the beginning.
>
> DENNIS: It was certainly less important at the beginning. But after we started investing all that emotional energy, I thought, 'Well, we can't give up now.' But before that, I remember thinking, 'I guess I will be okay if I don't have kids.'
>
> DORIS: You said that to me. You said it would be okay, but I didn't believe that it would really be okay. Because I am older than you, I figured that when *you* got older, you would wave goodbye.

When children are important to a man, his partner feels enormous responsibility for delivering the goods. After all, this is a woman's primary role, and it is being reinforced by the most important person in her life. He agrees: Yes, this is your job!

> Hal says, 'Look, this is the way it always was: I grew up, I knew I was going to get married, I'm going to stay married, and I want to have children.' He knew he wanted to marry a nice, Jewish girl and he ended up with me. And that is when the plan went a little bit awry because I am a DES daughter and we don't have a baby yet. So we have to get a

> baby because that is the plan. His aunt says it better be a boy because he is the last of the family. So not only does it have to be a baby, it has to be a boy!
>
> I can't imagine saying to him, 'Well, this didn't work, let's go to the movies and have dinner parties for the next twenty years. And then we will get old. And then we will die.' No, it is just out of the question. So we are going to have to acquire a child, and then it will be okay.
>
> —Marsha

RE-CREATING THE FAMILY

No matter how men and women approach the parenting decision—whether it is with boundless enthusiasm or cold feet, wanting to do it desperately or being iffy about it—endless questions arise as they try to imagine themselves as parents. Comparing themselves with their families and the way they were raised, they ask, "How would I do it differently? What would be the same? Do I want to repeat it at all?" In a sense, parenting is a re-creation of oneself. To undertake such a profoundly important experience is not only to do it well but to tailor it to our convictions.

Sometimes women and men want to re-create the family they came from. If they think it was perfect and it met all their needs, how can they do any better?

> We had the ideal family, the all-American family. We had everything we could want, and all the love. I had a close relationship with my parents. It was very family oriented, very warm growing up. Family is just real important.
>
> —Sally

But it isn't necessary to come from the perfect family—if such a thing exists—to want a family of one's own. Sometimes people want their own family because they didn't feel accepted in the family they came from. Laura, mulling over the meaning of having a child, said,

> I don't know the answer to the question I ask myself of where did I get this idea that nothing in the world was more important than producing life again. I'm sure this is related to the dynamic of my home when I was a child. My family's attitude was: 'Laura causes all the problems; she gets hysterical. If only she didn't get angry at her mother, or burst into tears over something her mother said, or her sister, or her father, we'd have a perfectly happy family. What is it with Laura?'
>
> So I learned to hold it back because I never got what I wanted. All I got was, 'Why don't you just stop that? We don't do that in this family.' I guess I want my own family where I can be me.

Not having a family to call one's own is lonely. It is like being cast adrift, without an anchor. If the family has been lost through death, divorce, or illness, there may be a strong need to replace it.

> My parents divorced after twenty years of marriage, when I was 15. I felt horrible about it. I still do. I think all children wish their parents would get back together again. I still wish that, and my mom is very happily remarried.
>
> —Sally

> It was an odd family. No one was very connected to each other. And now that my parents have died, everyone else has drifted apart. Since we moved here, it's like we went to the moon. So that's why I want to start my own family. People need ties.
>
> —Bill

Sometimes, children are more like parents to their parents. They become the little mom or dad. Parents turn to them for help, and the child takes care of them, or watches over brothers and sisters. When these children grow up, they may be in conflict, because they have done parenthood already. They may ask themselves: "Do I want to do it again? When do I get some time off?"

But if it was rewarded—if they were good at it, if they got a lot of strokes—they may consider doing it again. Being a parent is already part of their identity. So for them the question is not, "Do I want to be a parent?" It's, "Do I want to be a parent *again*?"

> I am the oldest of four. I helped my mom raise her kids. I was maybe more of a parent than a child to her in some ways. And incredibly resentful that she had all these kids. We were poor and struggling and had so many kids. Here I am, and I don't even have one.
>
> —Dierdre

> I feel a little robbed by my parents. I don't know if they wanted to be brought up by me or not. But it was my idea that somehow I had more responsibility than them, or as much responsibility for them as they had for me. So when I reached adulthood, I needed to play and not be an adult and not have kids—not be the parent because I had already done that.
>
> —Tony

If things went wrong in the family—things that can perhaps be fixed—then the wish to do it over again the right way may be strong. Repeating the past to get it right cleans the wound and heals the pain.

> When I was growing up my mother spent a lot of time in hospitals. I was the oldest child, and I had three siblings. I was in essence their mother. I felt like I was the maternal factor in their lives but was never given full responsibility for being their mother. I sort of played their mother. I really bought into that role. They were my kids. My mother didn't

> do a good job. She couldn't handle it. I always felt that when I became a mother, I would do it better. I was going to be a better mother than my mother.
>
> —Dorene

Regardless of what childhood was like, most of us felt anchored by our family as children. Now that we're adults, we want to re-create that feeling of being grounded, of belonging. Why do we fly home for holidays? Why do we burn up the phone lines talking to the sister who is still our best friend? Why do we get into the same silly arguments time after time? Why do we always have fried chicken when we all get together? Because we're a family. And as we get older, we want to re-create that experience—starting our own traditions and having our own touchy subjects. That's what families are for—to extend us beyond ourselves, to make us feel substantial, to forge the links that tie us to each other, links that cannot be dissolved.

> I think having a stable, common family life was a real anchor for me. And I felt it real strongly when we moved here, feeling like if I can't be near my family, then we can have a family of our own and we can put down some roots and really have some stability.
>
> —Susan

We plan things well. We get this set image in our mind of exactly how it will happen. But what if things don't happen exactly the way we planned? What if nothing happens? In Chapter 2 we look at how lives are affected when the body doesn't follow its script.

CHAPTER 2

TRYING

What triggers a woman's plans to parent? Most often it is the ticking of her biological clock. She notices the passage of time as she celebrates birthdays and anniversaries, as she graduates from school, finds the first gray hair, or receives an important promotion. These milestones of her life are reminders that time is moving on. Once she decides she is ready to have children, she usually proceeds in a deliberate way.

> I've always been a goal-oriented person. You know, one goal at a time. I had always put having children on the back burner, so after I finished graduate school, I thought, 'Well, now it's time to do the baby phase.'
>
> —Sarah

In their late twenties and early thirties, women start thinking about the long-term. They carry an internal rule-of-thumb around that says 40 is the cutoff point. Busily doing math in their heads, women compute the future:

> One of the pressures about getting pregnant isn't the short-term, it's the long-term. I'm 35 now and if we don't get pregnant for 5 years, then I'll be 60 when the child is 20. I think that people get too old for kids.
>
> —Rachel

> At 35 I think I will stop trying. I don't think it's fair to have a child at 40. That would mean I would be 50 when the kid is 10 and 60 when he's 20, and I could be dead by the kid's 30th birthday. That's not fair to the child.
>
> —Sally

Women think about the future and about growing old. They imagine themselves as old women with still young children. What will that mean? How will it affect the child?

> I don't want to be 60 when my kid is just graduating from college. That's a concern for me because my father was so old when I was born. He died when he was 55. I was four and I grew up without a father.
>
> So that's a consideration as you get older. Do you want to be burdened with a child when you are going to be retiring pretty soon? There's that to think of. It's real paramount in my mind.
>
> —Carrie

Women set deadlines that add to their sense of urgency. When a woman waits until she is 35 or older to get pregnant, like Laura did, her haste is especially great.

> If I do have a kid, I'll be 58 and still have a child at home. When am I going to travel around the world and do all these other things I really want to do? I'll be old, even if I can afford to do anything at that point after raising a kid.

Laura kept talking about her sense of urgency, saying to Stan, "But we have to hurry, I don't have much time left." In exasperation, Stan responded, "You're turning 40. You don't have cancer. You're not going to die!"

As women reach their self-imposed deadlines for getting pregnant, the deadlines change. The desire to have children overrides a woman's concern about doing things at the right stage of life. Women grow more flexible. Thirty-five doesn't seem so old after the fact. Neither does 40, if that birthday has come and gone. Women balance their need for a child against the rest of their life plan.

MEN'S WORRY: BEING READY

In contrast to women, men usually don't feel constrained by time. The number one concern of men is being ready. Suddenly, their name has come up on that inner bulletin board of assignments that we call men's roles.

> The idea of having a child is still freaky. Although it was always what I was taught I would be doing. When you get an assignment for something you haven't done before, there's a period of stress until you figure out how to do it.
>
> —Larry

A man goes down his mental list—a list very different from his partner's: How am I doing as a breadwinner? Will I be able to support a child? Am I ready to settle down? Have I done everything I want to do? Is this career going to last? What if I want to go back to school at 45? How will a child change our relationship? Will I get less of her attention? Will we both be sleepless and crabby for a year? Can we live in this apartment? Do we need to buy a house? A bigger house? The list is long.

But it's just as important as her list. Because this is what men are raised to do: provide for a family.

Rick described a scenario shared by many men when he said Angie took the first step. He was frightened of having children—he was just finishing graduate school and was not sure how they would manage. He didn't feel ready. Where would the money come from? They had been living primarily on Angie's salary. Having children loomed ahead like the Himalayas. But Angie said it was time to start, so he followed her lead.

> I guess I have to trust Angie in this. She says now is the time. She's always handled our family stuff, sort of scheduling our lives. And as time passes, I feel more ready for it. But it's a big step.

TRYING

Sometimes men are still ambivalent about starting a family, even after making a commitment to go ahead with it.

> I'm a little afraid of marriage. I think that commitment is an ongoing thing that you redo as you go. Signing on the dotted line lets people abdicate some responsibility for that. They go, 'Oh well, we're married. That takes care of it.' And I worry about not worrying anymore.
>
> But I guess I have to come to terms with it. She has laid it on the line, and I'd rather be with her than not. So it became clear to me that we're essentially married. And if we did get married, it would make the relationship richer, more committed. So we're juggling dates for the wedding around.
>
> This is part of my preparation for the next step, my evolution as a full-fledged adult with a family and children. And it's still shaky. I think that's why I haven't had kids before.
>
> My brother said, 'Have kids. Don't wait until you're ready.' But I *needed* to wait until I was ready.
>
> So I'm going to risk going ahead and not being totally ready, but ready enough. And sometimes I still have my doubts.
>
> —Tony

Men are sometimes ready to have children before women are, especially if the woman in question is petrified about her ability to live up to the task. But they seldom make it a condition of the relationship. Men don't have it listed as a duty on their inner bulletin board, so it's not loaded in the same way it is for women.

> Lou was ready much sooner than I. I never had been around little kids in my life. I had one cousin three years younger than I was, but everybody else was older and there just hadn't been any babies or any little kids. I didn't know anything about them. I just knew I hated baby-sitting in high school. I just despised it. I started working at a bank when I was 17, just so I would never have to baby-sit again. I was

> very, very scared about what was going to happen with our lives if we had a child.
>
> —Paula

GETTING READY

Sometimes two people don't meet and become a couple until they are in their thirties. And when they do, they need to give the relationship time to develop. And, in addition, each person needs time to get emotionally ready for children.

> I was 29 when we met and ready to have children. But he wasn't ready. So we lived together for a year or two before he came to his senses. Then we got married and started to try. I was a DES daughter, so it was a concern of mine. Could I get pregnant?
>
> —Marsha

As a couple inches toward parenthood, shifts inevitably occur in the relationship as they prepare to share their life with a child. Couples begin to anticipate the future. They redefine tasks, such as, "Who will carry out the housework? Who will take care of the child?"

The transition to parenthood is easier if each partner prepares simultaneously to become a parent. As the event becomes imminent, preparations gather steam. Couples buy a house, decorate a child's room, take a final adult vacation, change jobs, rethink careers—all these things happen as they make room in the relationship for this unknown person who is going to change their lives forever.

> We settled in here. We bought this house and started nesting, and things were feeling really comfortable. I liked my job and probably could have worked there part-time and had a child. It's the kind of job I've done for a long time, so it's not that challenging.

> What I saw was life change. Things that you could grab onto. A lot of creative things—projects, painting, something, anything. So I think that was part of it.
>
> —Dierdre

This is a creative time of life. As a couple, they seem to be expanding in all directions. They start anticipating the future together. It's exciting now that both of them are revved up. The child that started out as a question mark has now attained mythic proportions in their minds. This child is going to change their world. They are eager but ambivalent. They alternate between feeling at peace and worrying if they will be good parents. Now that they are ready, they expect conception to happen quickly. They think, as Cindy did, "One month. That's what I thought it would take."

TRYING TO CONCEIVE

Couples start trying. Some women get pregnant right away. And some don't.

> My closest friend and I both decided to have kids. I decided first and a few months later, she thought she would. Well, hers is about six months old already. It was just one month, and that was it.
>
> —Rachel

> I expected to just become pregnant. The first three months I went off the pill, when I didn't have any periods, I assumed I was pregnant every time. I had eight pregnancy tests that summer. They got tired of me at the lab.
>
> —Susan

Everyone expects their fertility to be there when they are ready. They just assume that once they remove the birth-control measures, their body will take over. Instantly. And if it doesn't, they are amazed.

> We thought we were really fertile and it would be really easy to get pregnant. We were pretty open-minded about all this stuff. Thinking that this is kind of funny because it's just a matter of getting lucky.
>
> —Dorene

For years fertility was a headache. An inner voice barked at the most intrusive moments, "Use birth control!" "Don't get pregnant," "Don't get *her* pregnant." All those years—of wrestling with condoms and diaphragms, of remembering to take the Pill, of wondering if the IUD was where it was supposed to be—have conditioned men and women to assume their fertility. All those years of trying *not* to be fertile.

> It had to come to marriage before I wanted children. I never, ever went without birth control until I was with Ned. He was the first man I ever skipped any birth control with, whether it was pills, condoms, diaphragm, whatever it was.
>
> —Donna

When conception doesn't happen quickly, men and women begin rethinking their fertility. They have second thoughts about postponing children. For some, fertility is an abstract idea. Women and men often don't know for sure that they are fertile—they have been so careful to avoid finding out. But they know it's there. Many women may never have had any health problems that led to questioning their fertility.

> My periods, they were always dead regular. I was always so careful about protecting myself—using contraception and not sleeping around with people too much. I was so sure I would get pregnant right away. It's all been a great shock.
>
> —Judy

It is even less likely men will anticipate a problem. Jerry echoed every other man I talked with when he said, "You never think about this as a man, that maybe you can't have children."

Most women who had a problem when they were younger usually thought they would get pregnant without difficulty—"because everybody does."

> I remember the first time I had a laparotomy,* and my gynecologist said, 'The best thing for you is to get married and get pregnant.' I just didn't think it would be hard. I didn't know anyone who couldn't ever get pregnant. You know, you got married and you got pregnant. You got pregnant even if you didn't get married, you know? I wasn't going to go out and marry just anyone in order to get pregnant.
>
> —Sally

WHAT'S WRONG?

Time passes. Women, now that their next job in life has become crystal clear, begin to worry. They start working harder at getting pregnant:

> Somebody told me to take my temperature. So I did.

> Somebody told me to put a pillow under my bottom after sex, so I did.

> Everyone said to relax. We would have wine with dinner and smoke a joint before going to bed.

> You get these statements like, 'Relax. Go on vacation. Go skiing.' We did all that stuff.

---

*Major surgery requiring an abdominal incision for the repair of tubes or removal of adhesions.

Men get into the act, too. Making babies involves two people. Two people and the most intimate part of their relationship—their sex life. At first it's fun, even exciting:

> We were trying very hard to get pregnant. It became quite a thing. You didn't want to miss a night of making love. It was fun, but after a while it got to be . . . It starts to wear on you. We didn't think of it in terms of a problem. So it wasn't that it became less fun about sex. Not that it is less fun now, but when you're first together it's all new. Not that I still don't feel those pitter-patters every now and then.
>
> —Carrie

All this work at something that is supposed to be enjoyable—and without results—makes women stop and think, What's wrong? They start to doubt themselves. Somewhere in the back of their mind, this little niggling doubt creeps in. A woman starts to think about it: "Something isn't right. This isn't the way it's supposed to be. I should be pregnant by now. After all, it seems like we're making love all the time. We've had some memorable times in the last few months—times that we expected to get me pregnant—the night we walked in the moonlight, the night we had a candlelight dinner, the day we celebrated my birthday. We went up to the mountains. Roaring fires . . ."

Women start getting out their calendars. A woman asks herself: "When did I have my last period? I'm sure I ovulated that week we were on vacation. Which month did we start trying? Gee, it's been three months. Four months. Five months. Six months. Something is wrong. Why doesn't he think there is anything wrong? Doesn't he care?"

Women worry. Men don't worry, at least not initially. They don't expect instant results, and their investment in a pregnancy is not so great—in the beginning.

> He has always been much more optimistic than I am. He says the glass is half full and I say it's half empty. So he

always said, 'You'll get pregnant. Don't worry about it—you'll get pregnant.'

—Paula

But women don't stop worrying. A lot of energy is being funneled into getting pregnant. Whenever we mobilize large quantities of energy for anything in life—whenever we invest ourselves in it—our identity is involved. The greater the investment, the bigger the chunk of identity propelling us along.

When things don't go according to plan, it casts a shadow across our identity. And if the degree of investment is unequal between us and our partner, we resent it. A woman may interpret her partner's equanimity as apathy or as negativity. She feels her efforts are being counteracted.

I felt like I was really driven. I became the primary force, and your participation was minimal. It always pissed me off because I put a lot of energy into it. Maybe it was that biological urge, that idea that I'm the one who has to get it done.

—Dorene

The differences between them—the importance of the pregnancy, and whether or not it needs to happen right now—begin to affect the relationship. Women start getting tense and jittery. Sometimes they jump to conclusions. If there's something wrong, it must be someone's fault:

JENNY: First I blamed everything on myself, and we had a number of squabbles about it. We went through a lot of blame. I'd blame myself and then I'd blame you. Wouldn't you say that was the time when we were having those, 'Whose fault is it now?' type arguments?

MATT: Oh, yeah. It was definitely 'Whose fault is it? What are you doing?'

Jenny, laughing at herself, said,

> It was either me blaming myself or I'm blaming you. There was a lot of blame flying around. And you kept saying, 'Oh, it's all right, it will work out, it's okay, you'll get pregnant, don't worry.'
>
> MATT: Yeah, I remember. Little did I realize that we were both infertile!
>
> JENNY: By that point I was sort of hysterical.

UNDERGOING A TRANSITION

When a woman does not get pregnant easily, she undergoes a gradual transition. It begins when she moves from viewing herself as not pregnant yet to seriously questioning *why* she is not pregnant.

> I was ready to say to myself, 'Okay, you haven't gotten pregnant in three months. I knew it was a possibility and that infertility happened, but I guess I really didn't think it could happen to me. But then I started rethinking those missed periods. I told myself, 'You're probably infertile,' which is, of course, unrealistic, too. So I think I began to react to it. And about the same time we were talking about moving here. I think all those things put together made it harder.
>
> —Susan

Women are constantly aware of their childless state because they want to optimize their chances for pregnancy. A woman wants her body to be a healthy receptacle for a fetus.

> I was always really down on those people who were just obsessed with having kids—that is all they could think about. I thought, 'Oh, how ridiculous,' you know? But you

> do get sort of consumed by it when you're not having any success. So now I've become one of them.
>
> —Rachel

Her perpetual readiness is reinforced by her reproductive cycle. But when her period comes, it symbolizes the loss all over again. Another month of wasted effort.

> When I get my period, I sit on the toilet and think, 'Go ahead, cry, this is the time to cry, you'll feel better.'
>
> —Laura

Susan spoke for everyone when she said, "You always think, 'This is the month. This month I'll be pregnant.'" The reproductive cycle orchestrates women's lives into a monthly cycle of ups and downs—anticipation and excitement followed by discouragement, depression, and despair. As time passes, this cyclic pattern takes on its own rhythm. And women become caught in it.

> Every month I expected that I was going to be pregnant. It was just horrible. Just devastating. I would get frustrated after a while. I couldn't stand it. I would have long menstrual cycles, and as time went on, there were some days that I would just explode. I couldn't stand it anymore, all the pressure of not knowing.
>
> And meanwhile, I'm sitting near the phone all the time to get the results of the latest tests. I wait and I wait and the phone doesn't ring. You have to wait for *them* to call *you* because doctors are always somewhere else. I just got frustrated out of my mind with the whole thing—sitting there, waiting and waiting.
>
> —Rachel

Loss of Purpose

At every stage of life, we are filled with purpose as the next stage begins to unfold. Always looking to the future, we ready ourselves emotionally and logistically for the next step in our life. We do this as we leave adolescence and again as we settle into our relationship with each other. This period of preparation eases the transition. We expect few surprises when we plan ahead, and most of the time we get few. Well, leaving adolescence may be a little rocky, but after that things usually even out.

When a pregnancy is anticipated and instead nothing happens, men and women lose their sense of motion through time. Their journey through life is interrupted when it is least expected. Life comes to a standstill when this momentous event does not occur the way it was planned.

> Life was just sort of chugging along, and everything was going well. We met, we got married, I had a great job, we had great friends, a nice place to live. Everything was just moving along. And then everything just sort of stopped.
>
> —Cindy

When nothing happens, women feel as though they made the wrong preparations, or didn't make them soon enough.

> I'm married, I've got a career, I've got an education, I have a condo. Okay, now we're going to start a family and nothing happens. What the hell do we do? What do I do with the rest of my life, believing as I believe? What am I going to do? I feel purposeless. I've always had a purpose. I've always been moving toward this point right here now. I've got what I want. I'm really happy, happy in my relationship. I like everything that's happening to me except for this.
>
> And it negates everything. I don't know what I'm going to do with the rest of my life. It terrifies me.
>
> —Laura

The sense of purpose—of moving toward certain goals as a family—is derailed as the goal becomes elusive.

> What you do is you grow up and get married and have a family. That's what you do. I've always pretty much had a goal in mind

> and stuck to it until I got what I wanted, whether it was school or my business or career, or whatever it was. So I got this far, and that's why it derailed me. It's like, 'Why bother to go to work if I don't have a kid to support?' It makes my work meaningless to me. It isn't working on people's loved things and making them beautiful for them. It's working on a bunch of broken and tacky stuff. So it changes the light of everything. That was pretty flattening for a while.
>
> —Donna

When life doesn't happen according to plan, we lose our sense of control over our destiny. We feel an acute sense of loss, that this cannot be. It's like a broken promise. It isn't fair.

After their initial surprise that they are still not pregnant, women renew their energy. They try harder. A woman thinks: "I can't let this happen to us. I must work harder at it." Her driving sense of purpose escalates. A woman becomes single-minded, as she puts all her energy into making the dream of a baby reality.

> I was real upset with myself: 'You know what's wrong with me?' I'd had an abortion when I was 20, so I knew I could get pregnant, but I didn't know what was wrong.
>
> —Jenny

Women's role as the primary person in the family unit responsible for the creation of a family leads them to initiate medical treatment.

> I realized that when I had children it was going to be more important to me than it was to Larry because it was going to affect my career and all these other choices in my life, so I felt like, well, I'm the one who wants children now so it's my responsibility to do this, to make the appointments, and to follow up on things.
>
> —Susan

For most women, there is a gradual shift in perception. They are concerned with finding the reason they are not getting pregnant. And they are determined to solve the problem. Most women seek medical treatment within six months to a year after starting to try.* By then they are sure there is something wrong with them.

*Infertility is clinically defined as one year of unprotected intercourse. Most books and clinicians use this definition as a rule of thumb. In this book, however, I define infertility as a problem at the point that one or both partners decides a problem exists and seeks help.

CHAPTER 3

IDENTITY DISRUPTION

> I identify myself as mother, wife, and interesting woman who does something else—a balance. But now without that . . . that's the hard part. I see myself as a wife . . . and my career isn't really anything. I don't feel proud of it. And so that's been a real problem. And I know it.
>
> And I have thought in this infertile, in-between time that if I was real fulfilled and had this identity with a career, then I think that would have made things a little easier because now . . . So as far as my identity now, I see myself as a wife, and as a person who is trying to have children, and now as an investment counselor. And I put a lot of energy into my job.
>
> And other than that, I go to the Y, and I have friends there and friends from work, and I go visit my family. So my identity is real foggy.
>
> —Theresa

The failure of fertility strikes at one of the most basic expectations women and men have for themselves—their biological potential. When this promise is not realized, the assumptions around which they have structured their lives suddenly collapse like a house of cards. Their world, and their place in it, is no longer the same as yesterday. When their world crumbles, it's like a bad earthquake. Everything tilts crazily in the wrong directions. And when the earth stops moving, nothing fits together anymore. They are left with a sense of chaos.

What causes this sense of chaos?

Each of us has an inner world. This inner world is our identity—composed of myriad images of ourselves, based on our past experiences and our expectations for the future. These images give us guidelines for living out everyday life. Our inner world guides our thoughts. It underlies our actions. It reflects the predictable, the comfortable. Like walking through our home in the dark—we know where the furniture sits. We know where the light switch is. Our inner world is like the well-known external world that we live in.

When the earthquake is over and this inner world is askew, men and women experience inner chaos. They are in a crisis.

> When you think about yourself as a healthy person and then you find out you are infertile, it really changes your perception of yourself. Which affects your self-confidence and everything.
>
> —Donna

How does this crisis come about? Things build up. Sometimes there is a sudden recognition that one too many things have gone wrong.

> Between everything that was going on with Jerry's job, and not being able to buy the house, and the baby thing, everything sort of built up. I mean, we came here and we have never been happy here. We have very few friends—I just can't find anyone that I really confide in. And he has never felt at home here. We suddenly realized we were in a real crisis.
>
> —Sally

> Having a lot of disappointments in our careers has made this worse. Because it was the last straw. You think, 'Okay, now we're going to live like normal people; we're not going to go for the glory.' And then it doesn't work, and you think, 'Oh man, this is really lousy.' That's why it is so hard.
>
> —Bill

Sometimes a certain event—or a series of events—triggers a crisis. Even if people have been living with a sense of loss, some events thrust them into crisis because they bring home the enormity of what has been lost. Theresa recounted how this happened to her:

> I think the low of this whole ordeal was last fall, and being at a family weekend. My entire family congregated at my parents' house. My newborn niece was there. My younger sister was excited about the new baby, and she talked all weekend about 'when we get pregnant; when I have my children.' I haven't told her about myself, so she wasn't doing it to hurt me. But it was awful.
>
> This was my other sister's child, and she was breast-feeding it. That was a real low.
>
> I remember getting away from them and just crying and trying to pull myself together. And thinking I just couldn't bear it. My heart was really broken.
>
> And when I finally could leave and come home, driving through the night and just crying and crying. It seemed endless.
>
> —Theresa

A crisis of this magnitude threatens the future. There's no looking ahead because the future is uncertain. To dwell on it is to invite despair.

> You've got to have dreams, I guess. I think that's important at this point. We were so dismayed with our childless situation that for a couple of years everything was just black. You could get enthusiastic about something for a few minutes but then all of a sudden the future would start marching up on you. And I felt like, 'What's the point of getting excited? We don't have a future.'
>
> —Bill

But there is no looking back, either. Nothing makes sense. All those plans that were made—they were made for a different life.

> So when this all came about and we found out that we were having problems, I was so devastated. This can't be happening to me, the person! What is going on here?
>
> —Dorene

When we realize we are in a crisis, we ask ourselves, 'Who am I?' We have to rethink the road map we made for our life. Where did we take a wrong turn? Is this a dead end?

> Finding out I was infertile made me question my reason for living. I had to find out who I was.
>
> —Penny

> The infertility has raised questions in my mind about the type of person I am. Unfortunately, I don't even know who I am, probably like most people you know.
>
> —Jeff

WOMEN'S IDENTITY CHANGES

When a woman can't get pregnant, it's a blow to her identity. She feels like a failure. Her identity as a woman is closely tied to her reproductive functions. She compares herself with all other women—women who appear to become pregnant without trying:

> As a woman I feel like such a terrible failure. It's bizarre. How can you have all these 16-year-olds who get pregnant by accident, who didn't really want to get pregnant? People get pregnant all the time. Why can't we just do that? What is the big deal? It makes me feel like I'm a loser.
>
> —Laura

> If every 13-year-old in the backseat of a Pontiac can have a baby, why can't I? And when I read about child abuse cases and all that kind of thing, I think, 'Oh, my God!'
>
> —Paula

A woman's identity is closely linked to self-expression through a child. The child becomes a symbol of the meaning of life. As the child becomes increasingly elusive, its symbolic meaning grows. For Laura, the meaning of having a child was bound up with the meaning of life:

> I'm sort of an existentialist about it. Life is meaningless without children. It's part of the creative impulse.
>
> We'd be a lot better off financially if I continued working and we didn't have a child. But what for? It's just meaningless to me. It would just be money. It would just be buying more things—window dressing to cover up my empty life.

When a woman is stymied in her efforts to carry out her purpose in life, she falters. She loses her way. She feels as if her very self is under attack. She is living a nightmare that doesn't stop upon waking. It seems unending, a torment from which there is no escape. If this is reality, then something is radically wrong. Everything about her—hopes, values, personhood—feels shattered. Donna described how infertility encompassed her entire life:

> I feel bad personally about not being able to do something I'm committed to. I feel guilty on the mornings I can barely get out of bed because my period has descended. All of it has given me a bitter outlook. It has wrecked my attitude at work.
>
> Mostly, as a woman, it's affecting me as a person, as a productive person. It's not necessarily the femininity that has been crunched but the hopeful attitude I've had all my life has been crunched. I don't know if I believe in God

> anymore, and if I do, I think He is a pretty mean guy. Unless karma is a factor. I don't know what I've done in this life to deserve this. I know Ned thinks it has kind of screwed up my values. But it seems like good people should get good things.
>
> I just feel like this walking wound, so vulnerable. So I guess it kind of touches on my feelings about my femininity, but I would say it's more a kind of drag on my whole outlook.

A woman may begin to feel that the way she fills up her day is inane. Pointless. She has always had a purpose, and now she may not be able to live it out. Life starts to stretch out ahead of her, meaningless.

> What are we going to do with the rest of our lives? Go on ski weekends? We don't even ski. What are we going to *do*?
>
> —Marsha

Some women feel so immobilized by the standstill they have come to that they feel as if they are dying, an inch at a time.

> Every month, it is exactly like a death. I remember when my father-in-law died. First I said, 'No, it's not true, take it back,' because he died suddenly. Then it's uncontrollable anger. Then you don't know what to do. Then it's hysteria and grief. That's the way it is every month. There is nothing you can do about it.
>
> —Judy

> My chances are getting smaller and smaller and smaller. It's like somebody has cancer and you say, 'Well, you have a 20 percent chance that you will live'; and then go down to 10, and then to 5, and then you say, 'You're not going to live, let's face it. You are going to die any day'; 'Well, you just have to give up,' and I guess that's where I'm at now. I haven't given up yet, but . . . I'm pretty close to it. I

> really equate this with dying. They say that not having a child is like a death. It's like having cancer. You feel like you have to fight until the last minute. You have to do everything you can until it's over. Until you are dead.
>
> —Sally

Once she is hit by a sense of crisis, a woman may feel tired all the time. It may be hard to get through the day. She feels fragile, vulnerable. Some days the sun is too bright, and yet it seems dark. She feels buffeted by the voices around her, like a too-harsh wind. People talk to her, and what they say seems meaningless. Who cares? Their words fall on deaf ears. She goes through the motions of her job, trying to concentrate. But abstract tasks have no meaning anymore. Very little *does* have meaning anymore.

Except for this one huge concern, this enormous weight she is carrying around. It has her total attention. It absorbs her with the same intensity a pregnant woman is preoccupied with *her* changes.

> I think I felt it more than Sam. I think he was able to sort of keep going but I really felt a real inability to be productive with my work life. I definitely had a less productive year. And I withdrew a lot from everybody.
>
> —Cindy

In her outer life, she is overcome by lethargy. She feels apathetic, inert, tuned out. In her relationships with others. In the daily round. While pouring huge vats of energy into this inner struggle. She feels as if she is wading through molasses, it is so hard to think. It takes a giant effort to mobilize her resources, to get through the day. She goes through the motions—of working, cooking, washing clothes, going to the gym. But her life is being lived in the interior these days. In the interior of her body. In the interior of her mind.

Day by day the outer world shrinks and recedes as she becomes more preoccupied with her inner world. She can't pay too much attention to what's happening out there. She needs to figure out what is happening within her first. In her head. In her body. "What was that? War in the Middle East? It's been going on for three weeks now? Oh."

She can't sustain this level of intensity indefinitely. Her life needs to take on a semblance of normality. When it doesn't, she feels as if this situation is getting crazy. What is reality? It's getting a little hazy.

Sometimes women anesthetize themselves—they shut down their inner world and try to live only in their body. On automatic pilot, they go through the day in a haze. When a woman does this, she is out of synchrony with herself. Maybe it doesn't matter since everything is out of kilter anyway. And sometimes it is necessary for self-preservation. But the jolt when she wakes up is severe. A single chink in her armor and she is suddenly enveloped in her loss. Marsha described what living in limbo was like:

> We are in suspended animation. Our place is nice and everything is in order. The jobs are okay. We go to work every day, we have our weekends free, we sleep late, and we do all these things. I started thinking, 'We have another forty years to do that.' And it hit me all over again.

When she loses her reason for being, a woman has to find herself.

This inner communion with the self is essential. A woman must do it. She has no choice. She needs to find some meaning in her life so she can reorder it. And to do this, she needs to search her interior. She can't live with this split in her vision—of how things should be, and of how things actually are. It is too disorienting. In this inner search, she turns over every stone, she inspects every crevice. In search of answers. Answers that will restore her life to her. Marsha was so intent on finding an answer that she thought of nothing else:

> We went for a drive, and suddenly I said to Hal, 'You know, I don't think I have thought of getting pregnant for ten minutes.' I think that's a first. And we started comparing

> notes. It seems like I talk about it all the time, and together we talk about it constantly. And he said he was thinking about it all the time. Yeah, I do talk about it all the time, and every waking and sleeping minute I am thinking about it.

Women gradually realize they are changing. Like Angie, they ask themselves, "What is happening to me?"

> It's right there all the time, whether I'm at my stable time in between periods or whether I'm getting my period. It's there all the time. I mean, not a day, not an hour goes by. I am literally obsessed by it. And Rick can vouch for me—I am not an obsessive person. Until this issue. I may obsess about family issues and things like that, but basically I'm pretty unstressed, pretty upbeat, just a goer. But this is really getting to me, and I don't like it. That's what a lot of people in Resolve* say. They don't like what it's doing to them as a person.

Where does a woman start to unravel this crisis of identity? She starts with her body.

THE BODY

Not being pregnant begins with the body. How a woman views her body—how it appears to her and how it functions—is at the

*Resolve, Inc., a nonprofit membership organization, was founded in Boston, Massachusetts, in 1973 by Barbara Menning. Menning was diagnosed as infertile and sought emotional support and quality medical care. Today, 55 affiliated chapters offer monthly programs, telephone counseling, formal support groups, and medical information to infertile couples. The national office, financially supported by Resolve memberships and sale of literature, produces written medical information used by chapters and members, a national listing of specialists used by Resolve to refer patients to appropriate medical care, and information on programs that perform advanced reproductive technologies. The national headquarters is located at 1310 Broadway, Somerville, MA 92144-1731, phone (617) 623-0744.

core of her identity. In preparation for motherhood, women go through a dress rehearsal with their body. A woman imagines herself as pregnant. What she will look like. What she will feel like. What it will be like when her breasts fill out and her stomach grows.

She starts healthier eating and drinking habits. She thinks about how she will cope with morning sickness. She wonders how she will get enough rest while she's working. She is already taking care of the baby. Preparing the site.

Rachel describes what this is like:

> There I am, not drinking very much, and not drinking coffee because you never know. Every minute I was afraid. I would go over to somebody's house and they would pour me a glass of wine, and I would think, 'Should I drink it or shouldn't I drink it?' It was just this constant worry.

And she thinks about giving birth. How she wants to do it. Whether to have natural childbirth. What about drugs? She imagines breast-feeding. Everything revolves around her body.

She reads books. And in the books there are pictures. Pictures of brand-new babies and mothers, flesh to flesh. She wants to look like that. Being the perfect size 10 is no longer important. She can't wait to buy maternity clothes. She can't wait to see her body change.

> With men it's not the same drive. They don't fantasize about being pregnant. Women do.
>
> —Judy

As a woman imagines all these things, she becomes focused on her body, attuned to its every nuance. Listening to it. Watching it. Waiting.

> You become so in tune with your body that if there's something just a little out of sync, the hope comes. You

> think, 'Oh, I don't have the same symptoms. I don't have the same pain.'
>
> —Carrie

She starts to imagine she is pregnant. It has become so real in her mind. It can't be an illusion.

> I would get all wigged out about when we were going to make love. And then, after that, it was 'I might get pregnant . . . Maybe I *feel* pregnant.' I would feel a sensitive breast or a little this or a little that.
>
> —Betsy

The Defective Body

But when time passes and she doesn't get pregnant, the way she views her body changes. Marsha, like most women who don't readily get pregnant, views her body as a vessel—an empty, decaying vessel. She describes her body:

> My uterus is bad and I think all my eggs are spoiled rotten, anyway. The pull date has come and gone.

The body becomes an alien force, an enemy. Like Sandra, a woman begins to see her body as a sterile, even hostile, environment:

> I have been asking myself, 'What am I if I'm not going to have a child?' I have just been feeling the worst one can feel. Feeling, you know, really barren and what that means, and what it means to others. That is certainly a very frightening place. I'm not really feeling like I have a leg to stand on unless I have a child.

Sandra's words conjure up images in our mind: Barren soil, where no plant will grow; an empty plain; the desert. Where does this terrible, life-defying imagery come from that a woman applies it so readily to herself? Where did she learn it? Embedded in our culture, it stares out at us from *Webster's Dictionary*, a thicket of damning words:

> *Barren: that cannot produce offspring; sterile [a barren woman]; not bearing or pregnant at the regular time; said of animals and fruit; not producing crops of fruit; having little or no vegetation [barren soil]; not bringing useful results; unproductive; unprofitable [a barren plan]; lacking appeal, interest or meaning; dull; boring; empty; devoid [barren of creative spirit].*

To think women apply such a term to themselves! What does it say about infertility's assault on their self-image? Whose values are these, that a woman applies so readily to herself? Are these *women*'s words? Do women really like and value themselves so little? Feminists have asked the question in recent years, "Why do women think they are nothing without a man?" A woman should also ask herself, "Why do I think I am nothing without a child?" Theresa, ruminating about this issue, finally said, "I don't want my only identity to be as a mother. There is still Me."

But identification with being a mother is a necessary part of the process when a woman aspires to this role. Because when women internalize a sense of barrenness—when being barren becomes part of their identity—life loses its meaning. Women equate fertility with nurturance. The ability to nurture others is central to a woman's definition of self.

Dorene's identity revolved around nurturing others:

> My friends at school, they would call me 'Mom.' I was very maternal with my friends. That was just part of who I became.

Ideas of women as nurturers span a millennium. They go back to the Greek myth of Demeter, goddess of the earth and soil, and to Sarah in the Book of Genesis. Back to the beginning of time.

These images have followed us down through the centuries, though we may have no awareness of this heritage in our daily life. But the images are there. They live on in a woman's identity. Dorene was adamant about her need to mother:

> I could not go through life without having children. I was looking through this book and found this quote from this unknown author. He said, 'Give me children or give me death.' That really struck me because that is how I felt.

A woman who sees herself as barren contrasts her body with the abundance of fertility she sees around her. She equates being thin with not being pregnant. It is the antithesis of our image of the earth mother who nurtures and envelops others with her warmth—a role women see as their job to fill in public and in private. Marsha's feelings of failure to live up to this role resulted in excruciating pain:

> I was at a big party. I was in a baby's room, surrounded by babies, and some guy said to me, 'You have this wonderful husband, a new house, a new car, so where's the baby?' I didn't even know him—it was like being in a Fellini movie. I couldn't believe he said it to me. And one of my co-workers was standing next to me with his pregnant wife, and his little daughter with bows in her hair was saying, 'Daddy, Daddy . . .' And everyone chimed in with, 'Well, next year you will be here with your baby.'
>
> And I felt so barren. I had on a dress that made me look real thin, and I just felt empty, like I'm never going to be pregnant. I thought, 'I am the only person in the world who is this *empty*.'

Not long ago, Marsha, like everyone else, was busy, full of plans, full of her self, of who she was and who she would become. A mother. Filled up, replete with the knowledge that she would soon nurture another human being. Starting from within her body. Excited about this giant task. A life work.

Today the world seems empty. She *feels* empty.

When a woman has these feelings, she thinks, "This body is defective. It must be. Otherwise, I would be pregnant."

She feels trapped in her body.

It doesn't matter if a problem has been identified or not. Maybe it's her partner who has the problem. Maybe no trace of a problem can be found. She feels the same way no matter what: deformed.*

> It made no difference to me that Sam was supposed to have the problem. I thought, 'I am this deformed, infertile person.'
>
> —Cindy

> It isn't easy for me to have an exam because I'm not straight, and everything is made for straight bodies. And the Dalkon Shield** really screwed me up. It just made hamburger inside me. I knew my uterus was over on the side because that's one thing that first doctor I went to did—he was always trying to straighten my uterus up and it was terribly painful. It was like trying to put your arm backwards or your knee the wrong way. It just won't work. So I knew there was something, a structural difference there. It's hard for me to talk about.
>
> —Donna

Until now, her body may have seemed like a machine. She took it for granted. She went through life, and it pumped blood through her. It produced new cells. It presented her with a period every month. Like a monthly report that the system is functioning.

But when a woman doesn't get pregnant, it seems as if there has been a systems failure. The machine isn't functioning properly, after all. If she has always been healthy, she is completely nonplussed, as Judy was:

*Women attempting to conceive without success experience failure whether or not they have an identified infertility problem, which is clinically referred to as an "infertility factor."

**The Dalkon Shield, an IUD form of contraception, was the subject of a class-action suit after it was taken off the market.

> I want my body to work. I'm disappointed that my body doesn't work, and I think that next to losing a limb or having a terminal disease, it's the worst thing that can happen. I'm just in total disbelief. I still don't believe it.

And if, in addition, her body image has always met cultural ideas about womanhood—what a *real* woman looks like—she may feel as though this is a masquerade. That she is just pretending to be a woman.

> This one woman said to me—I guess I was wearing a tight sweater—'How could someone with such big breasts not have children?'
>
> —Sally

She feels like a fraud. She is walking around with insides that don't work. They are hidden from view—even from her own view. But it doesn't matter that she can't *see* what's gone wrong. *She* knows that something is awry, even if no one else does. She doesn't feel whole anymore.

Like Marsha, she feels defective.

> The doctor was watching the screen, and he said, 'It's very small and it's *T*-shaped.' Now I remember thinking, '*T*-shaped uterus, get it out.'*

Sometimes the body seems to go berserk. It announces to the whole world, not just to its owner, that something is frighteningly wrong. When this happens, a woman feels like an impostor. Now everyone else knows her body is defective, too. Marsha, describing a disastrous ectopic pregnancy, said in bewilderment, "I had this accident. My body exploded."

Women want to be normal. Every woman wants her body to

*A *T*-shaped uterus is associated with women who were exposed prenatally to the drug diethylstilbestrol (DES).

function naturally, without help. She invests huge amounts of energy to achieve a semblance of what is considered normal.

> I want to be dead normal. I have this overriding drive that I'm going to be optimally normal on my own, and when I can't reach it, it drives me crazy.
>
> —Judy

Not only that, women want to *look* normal. Every woman wants to be the right size, whatever that is for her. Even though being thin contradicts the image of being a nurturing, maternal woman, being fat won't do, either. But women often feel fat and out of shape. And most humiliating of all, some women are even asked if they are pregnant! So being overweight is no solace. Not if it is contradictory to the image a woman has always had of herself.

> Then I got fat, and that bothered my image of myself because I'm chubby and fat. I lost fifteen pounds but I'm still ten pounds overweight. I can't bear to diet. What if I have a baby in me?
>
> —Donna

Rachel found out that efforts to create the optimal site for a pregnancy were self-defeating:

> I started cutting out all my exercise because everyone that I know who is completely out of shape is pregnant. So I figured there must be a correlation. Some doctor told me if you look like a long-distance runner, that will do it. So I stopped running. Then I thought aerobics—jumping up and down—would shake the baby loose, or even sit-ups. I didn't do anything. I got so I was afraid to move. Meanwhile, I could hardly fit into my clothes.

Just as bad, women feel old, because the failure of the reproductive system is a signal that the machine is running down and its parts are getting worn. In a society that celebrates youth—

where 80-year-olds look 60, 60-year-olds strive to look 45, and 40-year-olds want to be 30—feeling old is especially difficult right now. It's a message that time has run out.

When Sandra gave up running, she realized she had given up too much:

> I love to run. I run maybe five miles a day, and I've been doing this all the time I have been trying to get pregnant. Then I went to a new doctor, and he told me that's too much running, that it may affect my ability to get pregnant. So I stopped running, and it was just killing me not to run. But the worst thing was, I began to notice physical changes. I gained some weight, but mainly I just began looking *old* to myself. When I looked in the mirror, I saw myself aging. Then I felt even worse about myself.

These changes in how a woman sees herself affect her identity. She looks in the mirror and sees signs of encroaching age. Her inner feeling of youthfulness begins to dissipate. She tells herself, "I have to face facts. I'm not so young anymore." She looks old to herself. She *feels* old. Sally, 32, with hardly a gray hair or wrinkle in sight, said:

> All this trying to have kids has made me feel older. If we had had kids when we first tried, that was five years ago. We could have a five-year-old kid and a four-year-old kid, and maybe a two-year-old, too. You know, I'm old enough, I could have a 15-year-old kid now. But I'm old and I don't have a kid. Wrinkles, gray hair—I've got everything else.

As women experience these identity changes, they get reminders from others that having babies and being old don't go together. It doesn't just come from within. Dealing with this cultural message—that younger women are mothers, not us—is painful. Women feel they must respond to this message. They feel duty-bound to fix their body inside and out so that they look young. So that their reproductive ability is maximized. Women start to wonder, "Can I pass? Maybe I can now, but what about the future?" Women sometimes find that, while they may be comfortable with their appearance, others may not be, as Marsha learned:

> I've had gray hair and the hairdresser said, 'You can't be pregnant and have gray hair. Forget it. It is out of the question.' So he put a rinse on my hair. But I really do have gray hair. Now how is that going to be? These kids on talk shows resent their parents who are old. But they didn't *realize* they were old till they were teenagers.

Pregnancy is more than the sum of a woman's bodily changes. It is a state of mind. For some women, it is the only acceptable answer to this identity crisis. Nothing else can make things right. Pregnancy, in addition to all its joys, says a woman is okay. It affirms that she is a woman. That nothing is wrong with her, after all, that her body functions as it should. Everyone who has set off down this road wants to experience pregnancy. Because of the assault on a woman's identity, the need for a pregnancy grows ever bigger.

Marsha described how being pregnant reaffirmed who she wanted to become:

> I loved being pregnant. The old, preexisting insecurities and feelings of just being incredibly ineffective as a woman and all of those feelings about being big and coarse just melted away. I want to re-create that feeling I had when I was pregnant. I was only pregnant a month but it feels like a long, long time because it was imprinted on me—every nuance.
>
> Hal said, 'I've never seen you this happy. You will never be this happy again.' He was right. That is absolutely true. That is the drive. To re-create that feeling. The whole time I was saying, 'It's okay, Baby, I'll take care of you. Everything will be okay.' Here I was spotting. I had every

> reason to be concerned and frightened, and I wasn't. It was tranquillity, serenity . . .

No wonder women feel swamped by inertia when they don't conceive. No wonder they feel overwhelmed. When a woman gets a spurt of energy, she starts to turn outside of herself for some answers. She goes to the doctor, if she hasn't already gone. If she has, she goes back again. She has mobilized all her inner resources to get through this ordeal, to find some answers, to fulfill her life's purpose. She can't just give up.

She takes the next step.

CHAPTER 4

MEN AND IDENTITY

> It's hard for me to get inside her head totally—what her motives are—they change. But certainly wanting kids is a big part of her motivation. And I want kids. I would like to have kids around the house and to grow up with kids and to provide for kids and be part of a family with children in it. And sometimes she takes over with that, she's almost too forward with it, like I don't have much to do with it.
>
> It's like I'm always seconding the motion. And then I hang back. But I'm on the ship, too. I'm part of the crew here.
>
> —Tony

A man agrees with his partner: It's up to her to bear children. He may not have thought too much about the details, like who will change diapers, or who will clean up spills. But he knows one important thing: He knows this whole process can't happen without him.

Ability to procreate—to father a child—is central to the idea of masculinity. It is almost never questioned. Men are born with this potential, and grow to manhood with an ever-present knowledge of this promise.

His potential to father a child makes a man fairly nervous sometimes. He has spent so many years trying to keep things under control, an effort that started in adolescence, with wet dreams and erections at embarrassing moments. There has always been this unending supply of semen, no matter how much he masturbated. No matter how many condoms he has gone through. It has always been there. This is the emblem of his manhood.

He doesn't question it.

It's reassuring, actually. Because what if he didn't have this ability? This endless supply? This is what men joke about. Matt describes how cultural indoctrination about manliness occurs:

> The dirty jokes and the sexual insinuations in men's locker rooms of men not being fertile are just incredible. From the time you walk in when you are 5 until the time you leave when you're 25 . . . it really changes your opinion of who you are and how you view other people when you learn you are infertile.

Our language is full of words and phrases that reinforce this message—stud, hunk, jock—images of sexual potency. The word "stud," for example, carries with it a complex set of ideas about masculinity, potency, sexuality, and procreation. Who comes to mind when a woman applies the word "stud" to a man? A university professor? No. She thinks of the male centerfold in a woman's magazine, a quarterback on a major league football team, the last sexy man she saw in the movies. These are fantasies of the ideal man. Not real people.

It's not just women who have a set of associations about who can be called a stud. Men, too, have their fantasies. And the attributes a man identifies with this image may be more well defined: physical power, competence, wit, charm, confidence. Sexual prowess—capable of endless erections, ceaseless sexual activity, and intriguing sexual exploits. What a man!

Except that this is not a real man. He is some kind of cultural ideal.

Most men know this, but it is still our strereotype of what a man should be. What he should aspire to. This burden creates a lot of fear, a lot of anxiety, for men. Because every man probably carries some version of Matt's locker-room image around in the back of his head. So he lives with a fear that is perpetuated everywhere in our culture—that if he can't live up to popular ideas about manhood, he runs the risk of ridicule and put-downs. And who wants that?

Men are hobbled by this burden, some more than others. It affects how men relate to women and to each other. It inhibits the expression of feelings, of emotions. A man can't be "soft." He can't cry. He can't be "like a woman." He has to be strong. Hard. Tough. At least that's what the stereotype says.

Men vary a lot from each other in how much importance they attach to the stereotype. And how necessary they find it to live out the image. How can they measure up? It's impossible.

But men do attempt to live up to it, each in his own way. It's a cultural expectation. A man, in an effort to be realistic, may ultimately settle for being who he really is. But that image is always there, hanging over his head. An image just as potent for men as those prehistoric goddesses—women's original role models—that women have to live with.

Going back in time, men were thought to "plant" their seed in women. And a woman was seen as a passive receptacle, a repository for a man's seed. In some cultures, the idea of male infertility is inconceivable, even today. These cultures are based on the idea of paternity, a man's ability to father a child. This potential is not questioned. Underlying this notion is the idea of male dominance—that men are instrumental, necessary for things to happen in the world. This idea comes down to us through our stories of creation—Eve being created from Adam's rib.

Stories from the Bible underlie many of our traditions—traditions that say men make things happen. And in cultures that practice paternalism, men do. They have the upper hand. They hold the power. Paternalism is perpetuated in our stereotype of the real man, who is capable of anything. Feminist critiques of paternalism in American life tend to omit one critical factor in understanding the power imbalance between women and men—that men are victims of paternalism, too.

In our own culture, men and women struggle with issues of dominance and equality on a daily basis. We are in a time of shifting roles for men and women, headed toward greater equality—something men and women both want. Men themselves may feel that the idea of male dominance is outmoded and has run its course. Nowadays, they may feel there are much more rewarding ways to relate to women—as equals and as fellow explorers of the universe. Ways that don't result in role loss for them.

But this cultural baggage of who men are supposed to be runs deep. A man may be able to put aside the issue of dominance in his relationship with his partner. But it is not really possible to let go of the symbols—the central motifs of life—that stand for who we are. Symbols of paternity, for example. Especially if the symbol is a body part.

For a man, it's his penis.

A man's penis is at the center of his masculinity—his identity as a man. The penis and its fluid are the ultimate symbol of power and potency for a man—a legacy that has followed men down through the ages. A man can't just walk away from this idea, even if he wants to. It is ingrained in him—part of his fiber, the core of his being. His essence as a man.

It is the key to understanding a man's response to his fertility.

Because fertility has a different slant for men than it does for women, there is a subtle but profound difference in the way men and women view their bodies and how they live out this aspect of their identity in the outer world.

A man defines his fertility primarily in relation to his sexuality. And his sexuality is a primary means of self-definition and self-expression. Central to his sense of self.

MALE INFERTILITY

If a man has a fertility problem—if his semen has been tested and found wanting—his inner core of identity has been touched. His sense of masculinity has been shaken. Threatened. Someone has said his sperm are no good!*

*A sperm count of 20 million or more per cubic centimeter of semen is considered to be in the range defined as "normal," especially in the presence of good motility, although 60 to 100 million per cc are optimal counts. Harkness, *The Infertility Book*, p. 189.

> I'm very difficult when it comes to this. I've lost about fifteen pounds because of this. I feel very inadequate because I can't have kids. I'm sterile and I can't do anything about it. That's how I feel.
>
> —Jerry

> When I had the first sperm test, it was the first time that I'd ever had any indication of anything of that nature. And psychologically it was a difficult thing to deal with. So I spent a lot of time in the doctor's office initially. The infertility was upsetting for me.
>
> —Russ

Men equate virility with potency. These images have been confused with each other for so long that it is nearly impossible for a man to separate his sexuality from his ability to procreate. Male infertility has connotations of sexual inadequacy. Failure to fit within the range defined as "normal" in a semen analysis is akin to a failure to perform sexually in the minds of many men.

When a man's sperm have been questioned, everything about him as a sexual being feels under attack—from his sexual performance to all those qualities that are indirectly sexual, like physical attractiveness.

> When there's a problem getting pregnant, people assume there's something wrong with you. I'm sure it's on their minds—you know, 'he's too uptight, he needs to relax.'
>
> —Bill

Worse yet, a man feels emasculated by a negative semen analysis. Jerry, baring his soul, said, "What all these doctors are saying to me is, 'Let's face it—you're a eunuch.' "

Men see themselves as empty guns:

> All these years I have been so careful to practice birth control. Now suddenly, I come to find out I've been shooting blanks all this time. It's devastating.

> I'm a dud. It really bothers me that I have failed.

When a man learns he is infertile, it takes him time to acknowledge this crisis and face the unexpected assault on his masculinity.

> He has acknowledged that, 'Gee, if it comes to where I can't have kids . . . it's something that I never thought of, that I would never have kids, or could never have kids.' He admits that when he gets the final results it might be jarring or shocking. He doesn't know how he will react. To look at him, he is very healthy, masculine looking. So who would think, 'Infertile'?
>
> —Theresa

A man undergoes a complex emotional response that moves in stages from disbelief to anger, and then to feelings of failure and helplessness, and sometimes to resignation and depression. A man's response is similar to the response people have to natural disasters, major illness, disability, and dying—a testimony to the magnitude of a man's loss. A man may ultimately resolve his feelings about his infertility, but this is a lengthy process, involving months or years of rethinking his identity in relation to what masculinity means.

The magnitude of the loss a man feels is huge. His shock when he learns his sperm are not effective is so great that it's hard to accept, initially.

Jerry's irate response is typical:

> After six months of trying, Sally's doctor said I should get a sperm count, even though he had identified a problem with her. So I went and had one, then another one. They were low—they were like 10 million or something. I couldn't believe it. The whole thing is unbelievable. This infertility garbage—I haven't accepted it yet. I'm very stubborn.

Because of the threat to his identity, a man is often initially unwilling to accept the existence of a problem. It is recommended that men be retested when the results of a semen analysis are questionable or negative, since one semen analysis may not provide an accurate picture of a man's fertility.* Bill could not believe the results of his semen analysis:

> So I went to Planned Parenthood to get the test, and when it came back it said I had low motility. It gave us a very negative picture at that point, like, 'That's it.' Sort of final. It was quite a shock. In fact, I was amazed. I couldn't understand it.
>
> I thought it just couldn't be right. So I thought, 'I'll go back. Maybe that first test wasn't good.' So I went back the next day or the day after. And at that point the volume was poor. And with that, everything just went black.

When a man is forced to deal with an implausible situation that involves the essence of his manhood, he feels victimized and assaulted. He asks, "Why me?" He is angry. Indignant. The unfairness of being in such a position fills him with rage. The whole situation made Jerry feel wild with anger.

> And this urologist—he repulsed me. He said to me, 'You're never going to be a father.' I thought it was inhuman to tell me something like that. It really, really bothered me. I felt like strangling him.

The situation a man finds himself in reinforces his feelings of impotence.

---

*Most urologists prefer to obtain several semen analyses to observe the range of semen quality. See Harkness, *The Infertility Book*, p. 188.

FEELING DEFECTIVE

Sperm suddenly take on new meaning. They become tangible. Real. No longer taken for granted. And they're not that straightforward—they have all these different facets. It's their numbers—are there enough? It's their structure—are they made right? It's their viability—are they dead or alive? It's their potential to penetrate—can they get through to their target, the egg? It's the quantity of the semen—did there used to be more?

Suddenly, a man thinks of his sperm in a new way. In his mind he may see a slide with his sperm on it under a microscope. Dead. Deformed.

> I decided to test my own semen—I am a medical technologist—so I thought I would just quietly check myself out. I don't know what I expected to see but I was shocked when I looked through the microscope. There were almost no sperm! I was devastated.
>
> —Matt

It is always there inside his head. Something that was invisible. Something he counted on. His seed. He feels flawed. Russ, discussing lab tests of his semen, said in anguish,

> What gets me the most about the whole thing is the morphology. Do you know what that means? It means the sperm are *deformed*!

Deformities are disabling for the mind as well as for the body. A man thinks of himself as whole. Until he finds out there is something wrong with his sperm. When he does, his identity starts to change, as Sam's did.

> How do I feel about my infertility? It's a disability. I feel disabled by it.

Once a man begins to accept his problem, he feels helpless. He asks himself, "Am I still a man?" He is in an unprecedented situation. There are no guidelines for how to deal with it. Not only is it totally new to him, it is completely unexpected. Bill explained what this was like:

> Well, the issue of infertility never occurred to me until it occurred to me. I just never had any thoughts about it one way or the other. I never knew anyone who was having problems having kids. So the idea just didn't exist. But once it did occur to me, it really went through me. It was something that I just . . . It was a problem of a different dimension. I felt helpless. I still feel helpless. As far as my career problems, I just thought, 'Well, you're just going to have to work hard.' But this is a different situation. Because there is nothing you can do about it.

Russ was frustrated by the nebulous nature of his infertility and the lack of solutions.

> The problem has never been, 'You're infertile, face it, buddy.' It's always been, 'We can't figure this one out.' Sometimes a test comes out kind of weird, there's some problem here or some problem there, and other times it comes out no problem at all and other tests say, fine, no problem. There's no clear-cut answer. It's not as though someone's saying you've got a problem or you don't have a problem.

There is little effective treatment for male infertility. It's not something that is easy to correct. So a man feels his hands are tied. Efforts to treat male infertility reinforce feelings of helplessness and futility. Jerry, initially trying to hide his pain behind sarcasm, finally gave way to despair.

> So we tried some voodoo at the medical center for concentrating the sperm, all these wonderful things. Yeah, keeping

> your legs up, standing on your head, counting to 20 . . . we've done it all.
>
> The fact is that out of 95 million sperm, not one of them penetrated a single egg. This is humiliating for me, even though I have no control over it. I'm sterile and I can't do anything about it.

A man is much more likely to keep his infertility a secret from friends and family than a woman is. His shame is huge—it is so great he may feel unable to talk about it. And so he tells no one. Most of the time, only his partner and his physician know. Jerry was no exception.

> This really bothers me, you know, this outpouring—discussing all these feelings with a third party. *Nobody knows*, except our doctor and our shrink . . . And you.

His infertility is so humiliating that he may go to great lengths to prevent others from learning about it. When asked how he dealt with questions about infertility from others, Jerry said:

> I lie, I say it's her endometriosis. I don't tell anybody. How low. But I can't say, 'I didn't penetrate an egg.'* I won't, I can't do that. It's sort of a double standard. But I can't deal with telling anyone about *me*.

Men feel humiliation when attention is called to their infertility. Carrie spoke, while Russ stared at the rug:

> It was terribly embarrassing. It was odd for a man to go and get a Clomid prescription,** so we went together. Every

---

*He is referring to the Hamster Egg Test (or Sperm Penetration Assay), an older test of sperm function rarely used since the advent of intracytoplasmic sperm injection (ICSI), which is an advanced method of treatment.

**Clomid, a brand name for clomiphene, a synthetic estrogen also called Seraphene, is most often used to induce ovulation in women. This treatment is rarely applied to men today. (See Harkness, *The Infertility Book*, p. 194.)

> pharmacist in town wanted to tell us that it's a female fertility drug and why are you taking this? So we were constantly humiliated trying to fill this prescription.

Men inevitably begin to feel responsible, that their infertility is somehow their fault, as Russ did:

> And the problem with infertility is that in areas they don't know anything about, they throw up their hands. Our doctor prefaces every meeting with 'I don't know.' He is honest in that regard, and I can appreciate that perspective. But when I'm sitting in there, I feel like I've been scolded.

A man feels responsible even if his infertility results from a joint decision he made with his partner. Jeff and Sarah agreed on the vasectomy he had in his twenties. Ten years later, after they did not conceive following a vasectomy reversal, Jeff said, "You feel bad because you couldn't come through, like it's a personal failing."

When men learn they are infertile, they conjecture about the cause. They ask themselves repeatedly, "Why did this happen to me?" Everything is scrutinized in the search for an answer.

> Maybe I smoked too much pot. I don't think so, maybe I did, I don't know if I did or not.
>
> —Jerry

> I've been turning over this business about the volume in my mind. If I think back over the last five years, it does seem to have diminished. I guess I'm growing old.
>
> —Rick

Bill could not tolerate the helplessness he was experiencing so he conducted his own tests and experiments:

> I was examining absolutely everything about myself that I could and both doctors told me, 'No, there's nothing you can

do.' And I didn't believe them. I think I do now to a certain extent, but even so there's still something odd about it. I think to myself, 'Gee, I really wonder what is going wrong?' For instance, in my situation with the condition of the semen varying so much, I would rack my brain to try to decide, well, is it stress? Or is it lack of exercise? Or too much exercise? Or sleep? Or all these things? And so this month I made up some tests for myself where at one point I was making sure I was exercising, drinking very little wine, getting enough sleep. I got great results. The next time I did something different, I put myself under as much stress as I could. I altered the situation each time.

I got up one morning and I had to go and teach and it was raining and I really had the attitude when I got up that morning, 'Oh God, I can't get up today.' I mean, I'm always sort of a morning person, I just get up and go and do it. That morning I did not want to do anything that I had to do. I had to teach; I had to run errands; it was lousy weather; it was just horrible. And there was time involved because I had to do all this before the doctor's office hours closed and I was just feeling lousy. And I made sure I did. I mean, part of it was induced, but I really felt that way. And I thought, 'Okay, so now I'm going to find out it's stress that causes it,' which means during parts of the year we'll just have to forget it because I . . . there's just so much tension where I teach—it's seasonal.

But I got great results. In fact, even better than the first time. So it really wasn't a scientific test, but it was a close enough experiment where I proved to myself that these things really don't matter so much.

Which is good and bad. Because its good to know that you can live a normal life; you don't have to be in training. At the same time, it's bad because you realize that it's just not in your hands.

MEN WHO ARE NOT INFERTILE

What is it like for a man who doesn't himself have a fertility problem? If he doesn't, he lives with someone who does. And because of the global way a woman views her fertility, when there's a problem, the problem moves in with a couple. Like it or not.

A woman sees *any* challenge to fertility as a crisis regardless of who has the problem, because fertility is entwined with her whole life. So even if neither she nor her partner has an identified fertility problem, if she wants to conceive and hasn't been able to, it constitutes a fertility problem for her.

This isn't true for men. Men's lives are more compartmentalized than women's. So if it's not his fertility at stake, a man doesn't take it so seriously at first. It doesn't hit a nerve. At least he doesn't think it does, not in the beginning. It's only later that a man finds out a nerve has been hit—a nerve in his heart.

The issues for a man who is not infertile revolve around the relationship. So in the next chapter we take an in-depth look at relationships, and at a man's response when fertility is the issue.

CHAPTER 5

THE RELATIONSHIP

Everything was perfect. We had this enchanted life. We met and fell in love, bought the house. His business was going well. I got a raise. We had practically bought the baby stroller. We were looking for it.

Then our terrier died. It was really rough. I stayed in a cage with her for a week. I was so attached to her. I loved her. This was a real setback.

It was the first inkling I had that things weren't going to be so charmed. I'd always had the suspicion that everything I touched kind of turned to poop. It seems like everything I get involved with gets to be a failure. I thought I had paid my dues. I was thinking, 'No, no, don't let this start happening again.'

Things were all of a sudden not going so well. The doctor is telling me the same speech every month: 'Seventeen percent of all women get pregnant every month.' But it was never me.

—Marsha

Strain on the relationship often begins quietly, as problems with fertility eat away at the carefully constructed moorings that anchor relationships. Initially, a man reassures his partner. She's imagining things, jumping to conclusions. He's sure it will work out. But when time passes without a pregnancy, she becomes more preoccupied. And he starts feeling left out. He's resentful about it. He feels abandoned because she has turned inward, in communion with herself. She has become self-absorbed, enveloped by the fertility problem.

Women complain that men are not taking their fertility issues seriously. What about men? They say that women are taking things *too* seriously. They see a woman's emotional immersion in the problem as a threat. Polarization in the relationship begins here.

Loss of fertility *is* a threat to the relationship. As partners question themselves and each other, the threat seems to grow. As they become increasingly engulfed by the problem, they forget their similarities and shared concerns. They focus on their differences.

Men and women *can* counteract the effects of a fertility problem on their relationship. The question is, *how* can they do this? By understanding the dynamics that are involved. And by taking action that will defuse instead of load the marital encounter.

Part of this potential dilemma arises because women receive most of the medical treatment. They become engulfed by it, while their partner feels left out. These dynamics sow seeds for the development of mistrust. When a woman feels she is not being taken seriously, she becomes aggravated, then angry. A man, in response, becomes defensive. Carrie and Russ experienced this problem when she had side effects while taking clomiphene:

> The doctor writes out this prescription for Clomid and he doubles the dose and I start taking it and start flipping out. I thought, 'This is too much.' I blanked out, saw little white lights, had hot flashes. Now I know they are the usual side effects that you get.*

Russ interjected:

---

*Although they are often ignored medically, emotional side effects of clomiphene are common.

> I used to think this was a joke. I really did because . . .

Angrily, Carrie said:

> He was horrible about it—he thought I was hallucinating.

Russ responded lamely:

> I just thought it was a joke.

Carrie, remembering indignantly, said:

> I had high-blown personality changes. I mean, Sybil was my name!

Russ, still sounding doubtful, said:

> Then we got in Resolve and the other women started reporting similar things so I had to accept that it's a real situation.

A man wants to be part of what his partner is going through, but usually he doesn't know how. Because she has suddenly become an inscrutable woman. Hard to understand. He never thought of her as remote or hard to reach before. He never thought of her as temperamental. He never noticed she was so emotional, either. What has happened to her?

When he's mad at her, he sees her as a stereotype of women—what men talk about when they say a woman is being "a typical woman." Suddenly she's demanding, unpredictable, hysterical, and untouchable. All at the same time. What did he do to deserve this? He doesn't know what to do about it. For many couples, this—a man's bewilderment in the face of his partner's absorption in the problem—is the heart of the problem.

> Stan doesn't know what to do. He wants to do the right thing and sometimes when I'm really upset or depressed I get angry. I'm just irrational, and what I really want is someone

> to say, 'Hey, honey, it's going to be okay. Come here and let me hold you.' And that's not his style.
>
> I just can't let my grief out. I think it's because Stan has always been uncomfortable with that.

A couple's sense of connectedness with each other may seem to fade. Each partner feels unsupported, and in turn becomes less supportive of the other one. Rachel and Bill were overwhelmed by the tension and frustration that was suddenly ever-present in their relationship.

> RACHEL: We didn't handle the infertility well for a while. I was yelling at him and he was depressed. I think it put a lot of stress on our relationship.
>
> There was a period of time when nothing was right. I was all upset, just devastated. It was horrible. Bill was off the wall. It was all wrong and everything. I felt a lot worse then than I do now, don't you think, Bill?

Bill responded:

> It was just indicative of the frustration she was going through. We finally decided that we would go on a trip and get away from all this. We just picked up and went. We had a great time. But everything leading up to it was just too much.

Rachel described how the stress of infertility affected her:

> I would just get frustrated. There were some days that I would just explode. I couldn't stand it anymore. All the pressure of not knowing. I was a wreck.

Bill concluded:

> It's been really hard on our relationship. Nonetheless, I think we both feel much stronger at this point. There were times

> when it was pretty rough. In the beginning it was compounded by the job situation, living 2,000 miles from where we grew up, meeting new friends, dealing with the real estate, dealing with the weather. All these things. At first, infertility was just another issue. It became the last straw.

What is *really* happening in their relationship? This is the point at which their identities as man and woman diverge. As attuned as Bill is to Rachel's feelings, it's hard for him to relate totally to what Rachel is going through. Like most men, fertility, unless it is linked to his sexuality, is just not that central to who he is.

But it *is* central to who she is. Rachel, completely self-absorbed, is focused only on herself. She can't get outside herself long enough to relate to Bill. Her life revolves around her fertility right now.

POLARIZATION OF THE RELATIONSHIP

Differences between men and women are polarized when fertility is the issue. Huge crevasses appear from nowhere to open up underneath a couple's feet, creating one chasm after another. How could that person sitting across the dinner table, so well known and predictable, suddenly become a stranger? Celia described how this shift came about:

> Ron wasn't in favor of a work-up at all because he had a much more romantic notion of getting pregnant and he didn't want science to have very much to do with it. I was fairly impatient at that point, I think partly because I had this hunch all along.
>
> So that is when the tension began. We started to go down different roads. I wanted to know why we were not getting pregnant, and I was sure there was a problem. And he thought it was just a problem of time and romance. At that point we were on very separate paths.

Fertility issues highlight differences between men's and women's views of the world. As I discussed in Chapter 1, the different roles for which we are prepared early in life may have seemed insignificant before the effort to have children began. But once those efforts fail, subtle differences between women and men suddenly take on huge proportions. Each partner begins to focus on these differences. Although they have no way of knowing it, the differences they experience result from the conflict inherent within each person's gender role. These inconsistencies greatly complicate communication. They are almost impossible to tease out because they reflect cultural attitudes that are embedded in how we think.

The complexity of gender roles, combined with the need we experience in middle adulthood to finally evolve a separate self, results in an explosion, however quietly it may occur. That vision of a shared reality, once so mutually held, bites the dust. Before each partner's eyes, that single reality evolves into two separate views, as women and men begin to differentiate themselves from each other.

The catalyst is their fertility.

Whose Problem Is It?

When a man doesn't have a fertility problem, he feels as though he is the supporting cast for the central drama of his partner's life. He doesn't like this role. He feels as if he has suddenly been discarded in favor of a mythical child. The child they are to have becomes the competition, even before it is conceived.

The ambivalence men often feel about sharing their partner with a newcomer *after* the baby's arrival is first experienced now. Except, in this case, the child is not yet a reality. This makes it worse. The competition is still in the image stage.

He feels hurt. Angry. As a result, he gets detached. The intangible nature of the child makes it easier, though, to hide his feelings from his partner and himself.

A man often belittles his partner's preoccupation with her

fertility, hoping it will go away. Why does he do this? He is reacting to his own hurt feelings, and is at a loss about the best way to deal with this threat. Greg explained how he made the problem worse:

> I thought I was right in what was the matter with Gina and what was the matter with all the rest of the things. You have a problem? Let's deal with it and go on to the next thing.
>
> And, of course, the more problems Gina and I had between us, due to our infertility, due to our lack of communication, due to the perception of power imbalance in our relationship, the more blockheaded I became. You know, if it's right, then it's logical and you can see it. We clear this up and move on. Instead, it just got worse and worse and worse.

Under stress, we become stereotypes of ourselves. We cling to our basic coping style in an effort to weather the crisis. Greg got locked into stereotypic behavior in an effort to cope:

> Coming from a family like mine, you take on the aura of not righteousness but just being right. The element that contributed to how I felt and how I dealt with things was basically, 'Everything is logical. If it's logical, it's right, and if it's illogical, it's unclean, it's untidy.' And we don't deal with it. Because it's not logical and emotions are—you know—so illogical.

Gina interjected:

> Everything was black and white, and infertility is one big, fat gray area.

A man feels inadequate to handle his partner's pain. And he gets defensive about it. Could it somehow be his fault? Sometimes it sounds as if she thinks so.

> For me to be talking with him is . . . it's okay if I talk to him while he is reading the paper or watching TV—that's okay—but to talk to him with undivided attention is a real struggle. We just had a big fight over that. I told him I need one half hour a day, I didn't think it was unreasonable. He sort of agreed, so maybe we are making some sort of improvement.
>
> —Laurel

In contrast, a man who has a fertility problem suddenly finds himself in a crisis that revolves around the threat to his masculinity. But he may feel as though he has to compete with his partner for attention. Who has the biggest problem? Each of them thinks he or she does. And they both feel as if they are not getting everything they need from the other one. Both of them may feel so needy, initially, that there isn't enough sympathy to go around.

> There were times in frustration when she would say, 'Look, you're just going to have to handle your own problem yourself because I have enough to worry about of my own . . . this business with your semen. I don't know what to say, that's up to you.' Whereas before, going through all her problems with her, I would have to support her. That made me mad.
>
> —Billy

When both partners see themselves as infertile, they alternate between feeling at odds with each other and feeling united. Because it is *their* problem, and they both know it. There is a lot of stress, especially initially, but once they have both identified a problem, partners usually feel as if they are in this together. They are a team.

> There was a lot of guilt and blame for a while. It happened. Until we realized that it was nobody's actual fault. When you say it's somebody's fault, that means that they did something to deserve it. You may be able to say, 'Well, it's

> your condition,' but there's nothing you did to cause it. So you can't blame somebody for it.
>
> —Bill

What happens when a man is infertile and his partner isn't? A woman still sees herself as having a problem—she sees the fertility problem as *their* problem. But he doesn't. He thinks, "If it weren't for me, she could get pregnant. She could have the child she wants. I'm in the way." His sense of failure is profound, and so is his sense of guilt.

> We went through a heavy discussion, considering—not considering divorce, but we discussed it. The fact that we'd even discussed it was, to us, pretty far gone. He said to me, 'If you want to get somebody else to do it. . . . If you want to get somebody else . . .'
>
> I have never seen him so depressed in my life. This really killed him. He . . . it was like up till then . . . I don't know. Anyway, it was awful.
>
> But you know what? It's my thing, too. As far as I'm concerned, I'm as guilty as he is.
>
> —Angie

The relationship is affected somewhat differently, depending on where the problem lies. But the basic issues don't change.

Feeling Isolated

Men and women learn sooner or later that their view of the world is not identical. This discovery is part of the process of personal growth in adulthood. But when it occurs in tandem with the discovery of infertility, it may polarize the relationship. Shocked by their infertility and flooded by feelings of failure and guilt, women and men experience isolation from each other—one of the most difficult things for them to bear at this time.

The sense of isolation a woman feels is related to her identity and her feelings of failure to live up to her own lifelong expectations. She is extremely disturbed by feelings of isolation from her partner part of the time, and unaware of how she contributes to the problem at other times. Because of the identity issues infertility raises, she may become engulfed by the problem and view her fertility as a burden she must carry alone.

Laura's sense of isolation from Stan manifested itself in a recurring dream:

> For the first time in my life about eight or nine months ago, I started having a dream over and over again. That's never happened to me before. It was really strange. Not only that but the dream just seemed completely inappropriate. It didn't make any sense.
>
> Every single time in the dream, Stan would say very matter-of-factly, 'Listen, I just realized that I don't love you anymore and I think I'm going to be leaving. It's been real nice.' And he walks out and I'm going, 'Oh, no, please stop, I'll do anything, I'm going to kill myself, I can't survive, you've got to stay. . . .' Total hysterics.
>
> And I've woken up a few times with tears coming out of my eyes in the middle of the night. Then unable to get back to sleep again and spending the whole next day with a knot in my stomach, saying to myself, 'Hey, it was just a dream and the guy is not going to do that at all.' It's completely out of the question.
>
> I brought this up to a very perceptive friend of mine. I was just sort of joking and talking about it and she said, 'Don't you see what that is about?' And I said, 'I guess it's about my not feeling I'm a wonderful person.' And she said, 'No, what it's about is your infertility problem. What I hear in that dream is that you're being just tremendously emotional and you're so involved in what's going on. And he's not there for you. You really feel like you're alone.'

Men also experience isolation from their partner. Men tend to rely on their partner to meet many of their emotional needs. They have fewer approved outlets for social exchange and intimacy than women do. That cultural expectation about being a *real* man—fitting the stereotype—prevents many men from exploring the expressive side of themselves with other men. Before he can go beyond the boundaries that rigidly define who men are and what is possible in other relationships, a man has to work his way through a tangle of men's issues, such as to whom men talk and what they talk about.

> I can sit here and discuss it now. It's not something to stand around and talk about while you're putting at the last tee. I really didn't have anybody intimate to discuss it with.
>
> —Kenny

These limits on a man's social self means that he relies heavily on his relationship with his partner to meet his emotional needs. Since a woman is expected to be emotionally expressive and have a variety of social relationships, he may rely more on her than she relies on him to get emotional needs met.

The recognition that goals are different reinforces feelings of isolation. Theresa, describing the first Resolve meeting she went to, said,

> The guy that came the first night was there because his wife asked him to come. He felt that he could live without having children, it wasn't that big—I mean, he wants them but he would survive. 'I have my work and my fulfillments.'
>
> That was what Paul was saying, too, before he found out he had a problem: 'I think I can do okay without it. It would be nice but it's not going to ruin my life.'

A sense of isolation arises not only because of attitudes or emotional differences between partners, it emanates from within the individual.

> There are times I feel more distant because I get things walled up inside of me. And I don't know how to get them out without blowing up.
>
> —Paula

What can a couple do about it? They can start by talking with each other. When communication is ongoing, isolation fades.

Feeling Like a Failure

The pervasive sense of failure that both men and women express contributes to feelings of isolation. They feel humiliated by their failure to live up to their own lifelong expectations. Marsha felt guilty over her failure to meet Hal's expectations.

> Hal, his whole life, has expected to get married, marry a Jewish woman, and have children. So he got it half right.
>
> His aunt was right. She said, 'Hal, she has been married and has no children,' and she was right. I feel terrible about that but what can you do?

Carolyn, to her husband's amazement, offered him a divorce. Talking about it later, she said,

> He's the kind of guy who is just cut out for a family. It didn't seem fair to him. He always expected to have a family, and he could do that with someone else.
>
> He was amazed when I brought it up. We talked about it, and after a while I thought, 'What's the matter with me? This is ridiculous. We have a great relationship.'

Not only does a man who has a fertility problem feel like a failure, men who are not themselves infertile experience a sense of failure. Why is this? The myth says *real* men don't have failures. When problems begin to surface in the relationship, a man asks himself, "What is my part in this?" Greg felt forced to examine the way that infertility meshed with his general fear of failure:

> Failure is not pleasant for me and so affects how I feel about success. My upbringing was not such that I am very good at

failure. I wasn't prepared for failure. Failure wasn't really acceptable. It wasn't something you did or allowed to happen. So my coping mechanisms aren't very good for failure.

I've never experienced failure, been around failure, been in an environment of failure. It seems like a bottomless pit, a hole in hell. There are no stopping points in between, and there is certainly no recovery point. That same fear of failure is in the infertility stuff.

I know for a fact that I don't have any of the classic macho, 'I must bear fruit' type stuff—'my loins must produce the next generation.' I don't believe I have any of that, and I don't have any fear of sexual failure or impotence or failure to have offspring. I don't think I have that, either. So I don't think I'm driven. It seems to be pretty well contained in sports and business, classic male areas.

I can't cope with the failure stuff. When business goes bad, I trot that over and dump it on Gina and the can of gasoline called infertility is lying around and that goes off. I don't know if it is a detonator or the detonee or whatever. I refuse to say anymore what is infertility-related and what isn't, having learned that it is all mixed together like a fruit salad.

Rational Versus Emotional

The idea that men are rational and women are emotional is another cultural stereotype that crops up when fertility becomes a problem. This stereotype plagues a couple once it gets an upper hand in the relationship. Its destructive potential is huge. It may become one of the most volatile issues a woman and man face as they deal with their fertility.

Why is this?

The rational versus emotional stereotype puts men and women in boxes. When partners are mad at each other, they may resort to this kind of labeling. It makes them feel better. It justifies their stand, and invalidates the other person. They may say it out loud, or communicate it silently with a more subtle series of cues—body language or emotionally shutting down. Here is a typical interchange that is sure to polarize the subject:

> HE: Why do you always get so hysterical?
>
> SHE: I'm not hysterical, I'm just mad. How can you be so rational about something that involves our entire life?

Either way, partners know a label has just been assigned, and consequently, anger grows. The battle lines are drawn. This argument isn't between two people who are in a lot of pain, anymore. It has become Men versus Women.

When this happens—and it does happen all the time when the issue is fertility—watch out! This is combustible material that's being handled.

Like all stereotypes, this one carries a grain of truth. According to our stereotypes about who does what, men are supposed to be in charge of objective thinking, while women are supposed to be experts in feelings and relationships. It is true that men and women are socialized in these different directions. We are participants in—and sometimes victims of—culture. It's a cultural setup for conflict.

Looked at another way, it's a statement about women's and men's roles. Which is the better way to be? "Why, the way I am, of course." It's human nature for people to think that what they're comfortable with is the best way. Of course, the other person, who does things differently, feels irate and misunderstood. Suddenly, fertility isn't the issue at all. It has become an identity struggle—a personal issue—"Are you suggesting there is something wrong with me?" In other words, who is better than whom?

A rational approach to infertility makes a woman wild. She feels angry and hurt. She feels isolated from her partner. Greg's rational approach triggered a storm of reactions in Gina:

> In my family we were encouraged to debate, criticize, challenge. Gina's favorite word for me during our therapy was to call me the 'DA'—district attorney.

When men and women feel their relationship is threatened, their behavior often becomes a more extreme version of their usual coping style. For example, if he likes life to be calm and predictable, he may become more controlling. If, on the other hand, she is accustomed to expressing her feelings spontaneously, she may send her partner on a continual roller-coaster ride if she escalates her expressiveness.

This is what Stan and Laura did. They characterized themselves, respectively, as rational and emotional. When infertility began to take over their lives, they each took refuge in the coping patterns that had helped them to survive other problems in life. These survival tools, developed in childhood and adolescence, didn't work for this particular problem. Instead, the sense of threat that hung over the relationship was heightened. Laura became emotionally overwhelmed. In contrast, Stan clung rigidly to a rational, detached stance. As medical treatment moved into its final stage, he was still saying:

> The first thing to remember is that it's not my problem. I know I'm involved in it but I can't see myself as infertile. So there's that right there. I have no need to have a child.

When the relationship becomes polarized, alienation occurs. Personalities interact. Emotions escalate. One-upmanship takes over. Disagreeing over whether to explore adoption, Stan, frustrated because Laura was not ready to adopt, interjected a dig into their discussion:

> You haven't quite psyched to the fact that you could do this with some other children.

Laura, offended, became sarcastic and escalated the argument:

> Yeah, that is true. I have *all* the problems.

Stan, defending his point of view, responded by calling attention to their dissimilar goals:

> I have other problems. I had a horrible job search a few years back. So far this has been trivial compared to the job search.

Laura, recognizing that they have worked themselves into a corner they have been in before, but still angry, said sarcastically:

> Ah, the analytic man. The emotional woman. Strikes again.

Stan, stiffly, but wanting this argument to end before it got worse, responded:

> Yeah, right.

They sat quietly for a few minutes, then Stan, in a conciliatory tone, said:

> Yeah, it's stressful, infertility.

Laura, now trying to smooth over muddy waters, restated one of their basic differences that continuously got them into trouble:

> You go about things in a linear fashion, and I do things in this explosive way.

FIGHTING

> I am angry with Rick a lot, and I know it's because of the infertility. And Rick says it right out. He says, 'I can't give you the thing you want.' And it may not be his fault. It's nobody's fault, anyway. I have to remind myself it's nobody's fault.
>
> —Angie

Infertility fuels anger. A couple may start to have a lot of difficult, painful discussions. They may make strained efforts to talk to each other. Sometimes they feel isolated from each other when they try to talk because neither one can see the other's viewpoint.

Or a man may not want to talk about it. He feels so inadequate. What can he say? "Don't worry. It will be all right. It won't take much longer, you'll see." He's already said that many times, and now she gets mad if he says it.

When they fight, she often cries and says he is insensitive. And he has been trying so hard to support her. And not getting any attention himself.

> She makes me feel like a creep! It's not my fault. I was just trying to be logical.

Sometimes anger seems to come out of nowhere. It becomes displaced and flies around like a poltergeist, causing unexpected havoc in daily life. Angie found that the simplest encounters with Rick became complex:

> It just gets tiresome. He came home for lunch today, and he was not even coming home for lunch, he was just coming home for something. And I should be glad to see him, and I wasn't glad to see him. He could tell, and it pissed him off. I said, 'When are you going to come back?' And he said, 'I don't know.' He was real mad, and finally I apologized. I said, 'I'm sorry, I just feel crabby.' And he knew it. I don't know . . . little things set me off. I don't even know if today was fertility-related. Some stupid thing sets me off and then I blame him. And he does the same thing to me.

Feelings that are first raised in infertility treatment are not contained in medical care. They spill over to contaminate other aspects of the relationship. Months after Russ and Carrie had learned about the option of donor insemination (DI),* it was still

*Donor insemination (DI), the use of sperm from someone other than a woman's partner for the purpose of achieving pregnancy.

an emotionally loaded topic. Remembering the shock they had each felt at the discovery of Russ's infertility, their voices rose in anger as they remembered a meeting with their doctor differently:

> RUSS: AID came up right from the beginning. He made us aware of what it was and that there was a donor clinic, and we should seriously consider that.

> CARRIE: I think you're wrong about that. He has and he hasn't. He hasn't pushed that on anybody. I've been pursuing that.

> RUSS: I don't think you're characterizing this very correctly because I was extremely upset by what I felt was a high degree of pressure toward donor insemination.

In a more conciliatory tone, he added:

> I'm ready to do it now but I wasn't ready then.

Personality differences between Paula and Lou were magnified and added friction to their daily life:

> Lou has one really strong characteristic and that is that he bugs and bugs and bugs until he finds out what is wrong. He never lets a snitty mood go by. I mean, he'll let it go by for a day because everybody can have a bad mood, but he senses when there's something really there. That lingers, then he is just after it until there is a total confrontation and it all comes out.
>
> And I tend to push things down inside like Scarlett O'Hara. 'I'll think about it tomorrow.' Until I get overwhelmed, and then I get totally unglued.

Sometimes people become afraid to fight. They hold things in because they are afraid an argument will escalate too far, and then they will have to live with the consequences.

> We fight like crazy sometimes. We are passionate people. We have horrible fights. We can really hurt each other, and yet he knows I love him and I know he loves me.
>
> Actually, we have not fought as much since the infertility thing really started. I would say in the last six months we have not fought as much. We usually have a good fight every month. Like a period.
>
> —Angie

Angie realized that fighting may threaten the relationship when there is a fertility problem:

> I think fighting gets dangerous when there's infertility. It gets very ugly. I remember a fight when we were first going through infertility. . . . I do partly credit him with the fact that we haven't fought as much. I think he is growing up.

Laughing, she added:

> I'm already grown up, of course.

In a more thoughtful tone, she continued:

> We will probably always have fights but they are not good for us. Sometimes our fights are unhealthy. We are emotionally interdependent. He meets all my needs. If we fight, I can't call up other people. He *is* the other people.

She reflected on how she thought their relationship would be affected in the long run:

> It has definitely affected our relationship. There is no question. I don't think it has made us love each other any less. I know we will resolve things. I am not worried about that. It is just something else we have to work on. I know we will deal with it.
>
> I think I understand it all. It's not something that I am

> scared about for our relationship. I'm not scared that the infertility is going to break us up. It has brought us closer. It really has. We both feel the same way about it. But it is a big concern to both of us.

SEX

A couple's sexual relationship is one of the greatest potential sources of intimacy they have together. When life starts to feel as if it is falling apart, men and women want to take refuge in their intimacy. But often they can't retreat into sex together. There is no solace to be found in sex anymore because infertility invariably affects the sexual relationship. Sex, already laden with emotion and symbolic meaning for a couple, now acquires other layers of meaning that revolve around stigma, illness, and the failure to conceive. When a couple's sexual relationship suffers, the threat to the relationship becomes a serious concern.

> At first we were dealing with the infertility. But then we stopped taking it in stride. We both got real depressed and we would get angry. It doesn't do a lot for your sex life. You ask yourself, 'Why go to bed? What for?'
>
> —Dierdre

Women and men become resentful when infertility interferes with sex:

> Our sex life has gotten really rotten because you can't make love after you ovulate because you might shake loose an egg that is trying to implant. And I don't want to during my period because I feel lousy. So there is just this little bit of time, and you have to do it right now, tonight, and you just don't have a choice.
>
> Sex used to be just perfect for Ned and me. Both of us, we were the most satisfied. He was the most satisfying

> partner I've ever been with. So infertility has wrecked that for me and I resent that.
>
> —Donna

Donna, full of angry frustration over infertility wrecking her sex life with Ned, has her facts wrong—important facts that are further damaging their sexual relationship. It's a fallacy that a couple can't make love after ovulation. In fact, it's a fallacy guaranteed to put tremendous stress on the marital relationship. The truth is, couples can make love anytime they want to. Intercourse is not going to interfere with the fertilization process or the budding of a fetus.

The primary deterrent to sex has nothing to do with physiology—it's emotional. Women may lose interest in sex because it has become loaded with feelings of failure and despair. Sex may no longer be for enjoyment in a woman's mind. It isn't lighthearted, it isn't an occasion for happiness or intimacy. Sex has become tinged with sadness. She may feel apathetic. She may fight off tears.

Sex has become work for her—a job—one she feels she is failing at miserably. Because of a woman's lifelong training to seek out continuity in her life, she can't compartmentalize her head and just live in the moment. Sex has become another symbol of her inadequacy as a woman.

> We go to bed often because we have to, but lately I'm not interested. When I am interested, I am really interested, but I'm just not very interested in sex right now.
>
> —Angie

> The quality of sex is different five years after infertility starts. The problem with sex remains longer than other problems. Women's enjoyment of sex is harder to come by because of all those feelings being there. I'm sure it's not just me.
>
> —Penny

Here lies another difference between women and men. Women's feelings—about themselves and about the situation—

interfere with their ability to separate their sexuality from their fertility. But a man funnels much of his emotional expression through his sexuality. This goes back to the cultural emphasis on sexuality as a symbol of a man's identity. Sex may be more important to him than ever right now.

What happens when a man lives out much of his expressive side in his sexual relationship, and suddenly his partner has lost interest? Sex becomes charged. She may not be enjoying it right now. Maybe she has said so. Maybe she has said it's a reminder of her sense of failure. Even if she hasn't said anything, maybe it's obvious to him, anyway. Sex has turned into a business conference for egg and sperm to meet. It is dead serious. They may both feel performance pressure.

> In terms of our sex life, for a week out of the month sex was purely mechanical. Actually, we kept saying this fall, 'If only we had insulated the bedroom before now. Our upstairs is now 20 degrees warmer and Lou said, 'Why didn't we do this last year when we were freezing to death, screwing at one o'clock in the morning?' You know, practically dying because it was 40 degrees in this bedroom. Now that I'm pregnant and we don't need to screw, we have insulated the house!
>
> —Paula

Couples are often at a loss to defuse a situation that is growing more difficult with each passing month. What can they do about it? They can start by talking about their sex life. And if they keep talking about it, they will at least *know* what their partner is thinking and feeling, instead of guessing.

And, just as important, talking about sex fosters emotional intimacy. Paula and Lou resorted to humor. It helped.

> I guess humor got us through that week. There can't be anything terribly passionate about him climbing off an airplane at ten at night and having this very short period of time before he had to fly off to another conference. Neither

> of us was very excited about it. I really missed spreading it out and having a nicer time with it all.

Penny and George, who had conceived a child after a lengthy infertility work-up, were working on having a second child.*

> There's a time period in which you are supposed to have intercourse. It's like a window. You have to make an appointment for it. I'm going to be home at six-thirty tonight so we can get our son to bed. Tomorrow morning I have to go in late and all that kind of stuff.
>
> It was very depersonalizing—to have to go get ready to make love and do what we have to do—it was just making things worse.
>
> —George

If that time period has lost its sexual appeal, it may help to compartmentalize that week, to have fewer expectations for it than for the rest of the month. Otherwise, the regimentation and the businesslike aura of this appointment may begin to engulf all the other times, the times it doesn't need to be like this.

Both partners may feel a lot is missing in sex—maybe all of the expressions of care and feeling that usually accompany it. A man resents this. It reinforces his feelings of being abandoned, uncared for. He isn't getting his needs met. And he may not be able to put his finger on exactly what is missing. But he knows something is. And the crazy thing is, he feels guilty!

Rick knew Angie had lost interest in sex. She said so. And her orgasms were infrequent, to prove it. To complicate matters, he was the one who had a fertility problem, but he hadn't lost interest in sex. If men who have a fertility problem have any loss of interest in sex, it's probably temporary, during the initial shock of learning they have a problem. But interest in sex usually returns fairly soon. Except now it is loaded—loaded with feelings of

*Secondary infertility is the inability to conceive and give birth to another child after one or more successful pregnancies.

inadequacy. Loaded with feelings of "Will she still want me?" Loaded with the need to express intimacy and caring in this traditional masculine way. And loaded with the need to perform—to please her—more than ever.

It's a no-win situation. Because by this time most women have gone too far inside themselves to meet their partner's needs and respond in a way he will find satisfying.

> As far as orgasms or anything like that, I'm just not that interested. And Rick feels terrible about it. He wants me to be satisfied for his ego. And he wants to be satisfied, too.
>
> We had a big fight a few months ago that really affected our relationship. It definitely affected our sexuality. There is no question. He feels that now there is a question about his sperm count, it's in bed with us every time we are in bed together. There it is, every time.
>
> —Angie

Sometimes anger becomes explosive. When it does, it endangers the sexual relationship. Laura described what happened to her and Stan:

> All the things you read about—that men feel like they are just a tool. You have to have an erection and ejaculate at a certain time whether you want to or not. He has said to me in times out of genuine anger, 'I feel like all you want me for is to make a baby. You don't really want me, you just want me to do it.'
>
> And that was real hard for me to hear because I'm so involved in trying to hold myself together, and Stan keeps everything so much to himself that I hadn't noticed this was happening. We had a couple of real battles about it, and we've had a lot of sexual trouble. We just virtually don't have a sex life anymore.
>
> Because we failed several times, and I do say, 'we.' It was him a couple of times and once I was just so uptight he couldn't enter me. I knew it, I could just feel it. I just

couldn't get relaxed. And I think the first time he failed, I just exploded. I mean a terrible explosion.

I didn't get angry with him, I just showed anger, and I can't even remember the dynamic. It was one of the worst fights we have ever had. I remember I waited until he left the house and then I really exploded. I made sure the people downstairs weren't home and then I just screamed and yelled and ranted and raved at the walls.

Anger expressed during sex can have long-term repercussions.

After that he was really angry, really resentful, and he didn't want any sex. He was withholding. He wanted to withhold himself because he felt like he was being used, prostituted. At that point I sat down and had a big, serious talk with myself and said, 'Hey, look, let's pretend you were him for a change.' Yeah, absolutely, it must be just awful. All I have to do is relax. He has to get hard and stay hard and do it.

So I decided I was going to shut up, and I would go along with what he wanted to do in exchange for his willingness to perform when I ovulate. He told me that, frankly, he just didn't like sex right now. He didn't want it. He associated intercourse with failure and stress. I did too, very much.

I thought to myself, 'Okay, this isn't going to go on forever.' I mean, we are either going to get pregnant, or we are going to adopt, or we are not going to have children. But for now I'm just going to go with what he wants.

They altered their sexual relationship in an effort to get through the infertility work-up without more crises:

What we seem to have gotten to on a real low-key and infrequent basis is sex without intercourse, which is a real relief to him. It's a real relief to both of us. I don't have to worry about, 'Am I lubricated?' He doesn't have to worry, 'Am I hard?' and we both enjoy it.

When Laura and Stan's sex life got derailed, it affected their medical treatment.

> That time I had to call the doctor's office and say, 'Is there anything that can be done to save the month? This is just so stressful.' She said, 'Well, I think he could send in a sperm sample.' I said, 'You're kidding. Why didn't you tell me that before?' And do insemination, which is actually what we have done since then.* It was a tremendous relief to both of us.

But by then the damage was done.

Her sense of failure was reinforced by the knowledge that another person knew:

> Before all this happened, my doctor said to me, 'Don't let me see on your chart what I see on a lot of women's charts, lots of little marks for sex around ovulation time and a total blank the rest of the time. Don't let sex become just for procreation.'
>
> That was before we failed. So I have been putting arrows for nonexistent sex for months, saying to myself maybe I should tell him the truth because maybe it's affecting the sperm's motility.
>
> Once I said to him I was having a hard time relaxing—maybe it was after the time I was just too tight. I had to cancel a postcoital test,** and he said to me he was hearing I was having sexual problems. And I can't talk to him about it—I just start to cry, and I can't stop. Now that he knows, my sense of failure about this is even worse.

There are ways to avoid a catastrophe like this. Part of the answer lies in defusing things before anger gets explosive. Not

*Artificial insemination by husband (AIH) is usually done to bypass cervical mucus that is inhospitable to sperm.

**The postcoital test observes the quality of midcycle cervical mucus and the sperm's reaction to it.

buying into the men versus women mind-set is one way. Using humor is another. A third way is to talk about it and together explore other ways of expressing the love and caring that was once so much a part of the sexual relationship—*before* it lies in tatters at a couple's feet.

But there are other ways as well. In subsequent chapters we will explore the various ways couples work to create unity in the relationship. Ways that can transform the relationship for the better.

CHAPTER 6

FACING THE WORLD

Once women and men start to ask themselves, "What's wrong with me?" life gets more complicated. They usually don't want anyone to know that they're trying. Or that it is becoming a big deal. Why not?

> I think the secrecy is tied up with our feelings about sexuality. Because I think most people connect fertility with virility, for men, and what is it with women—fecundity? I think in this culture success is measured by a person's sexuality. I know that's a lot of it for me, that there must be something wrong with me, that this is what I am being punished for. That if I had it all together this wouldn't be happening. That I'm not warm enough sexually. Although I know a lot of cold women who have a lot of children. I mean, my mother!
>
> —Angie

No matter how lack of success is interpreted, women feel inadequate. They say nothing because not getting pregnant has become a sore spot, a red flag. An announcement that there is something wrong.

Women and men find themselves feeling sensitive about a whole range of subjects—fertility, motherhood, fatherhood, sexuality—subjects that are cultural symbols for what men and women do at this time of life. Anything that brushes up against their identity feels like an assault with a Mack truck—topics that wouldn't have fazed them last year or even six months ago.

Lisa described how she felt when her infertility was publicly acknowledged:

> My husband is much more open than I am. He told people at work we were trying. So we were at the office Christmas party, and I was talking with this older couple, and right in the middle of what I was saying, just totally unrelated, this man burst out with, 'Oh, honey, my wife and I are praying for you.'
>
> I was just floored. And then I stopped to think, 'How are the rest of the people here looking at us?' We can't just be a couple here like everyone else. They don't know what it's like. They were just ignorant. They had grown children, and they were just being nice.

Situations like this keep cropping up. It's like an invisible wall. Just going along, minding one's business, suddenly, like Lisa, we walk into it. This wall is the culture. It can't be seen, it can't be touched, but it's everywhere. And it springs up at the most awkward moments. Just when everything is going okay. Just when it seems as if the idea that something is wrong is just a silly notion—that's the moment—the moment when things fall apart. The moment we feel put on the spot, our face turns red, we break out in a stammer. The moment we wished we had stayed home. "Oh no, here it is *again*." At parties, baby showers, summer barbecues. At weddings, right after toasting the bride and groom. At family get-togethers. Everywhere.

Marsha, talking about a party she went to, where her infertility became public knowledge, said:

> Somebody standing in this circle of people said, 'Well, she's trying.' I couldn't believe it. I started to feel real light-headed, you know, dizzy with the intensity of it. I felt singled out, like I was the only one in the world without a child. And I just walked out . . . in a daze.

We leave these encounters feeling that we are "the only one in the world." In other words, we feel *different* from others. No longer their equal. As Bill said,

> If you're infertile, you know the meaning of stigma because it makes you different from everyone else.

THE STIGMA OF INFERTILITY

When we feel we can't live up to cultural expectations about what is normal, we experience stigma. We *do* feel different from others in a very specific way—that we are somehow not as good as they are. A stigma is a blemish, a moral taint.

> The first thing people ask you is how many children you have. We get it all the time. And we say, 'None.' And they go, 'Huh.' As though to say, 'What's the matter with you? Don't you like kids? What are you, a Nazi or something?
>
> —Jerry

How women and men feel about themselves reflects how they view their fertility and how they imagine others will view them if the truth becomes known. In this process of comparing oneself with others, the inability to conceive gradually blights everything, even social encounters with strangers. Why do these situations take such a personal toll? A person feels devalued when a private stigma threatens to become public knowledge. At moments like this, we see ourselves through others' eyes. And, as a result, our identity is permanently affected.

> RACHEL: We work in the same place. We are negotiating a new contract at work and I wanted to make sure there would be some kind of leave for people who adopt. That was my idea. I don't think I should be penalized because I get this little baby and I didn't have it naturally, if everyone else gets six weeks off and I have to go back to work the next day. That is ridiculous. So that meant talking to people on the committee negotiating the contract, and they've got big mouths. Before you know it, the whole committee knows.

> And there is one woman on there, if she knows something, the whole office knows.

> BILL: Well, we knew everyone knew because people in the department started saying things to us. One guy said to me, 'Get those sex books out and study them.' You know, the insinuation is that we don't know how to do things right and that is why we are not getting pregnant. Just totally ignorant statements like that are really bothersome. Although I don't think it's malicious.
>
> The thing that bothers me is not what they think of me but their ignorance and lack of understanding. I feel a stigma like infertility is nobody's business, because they are not going to understand. Yet it has to be their business if they are in the position of making decisions.
>
> So that's what makes it difficult. It's so weird that you have to take somebody aside in confidence and sort of educate them about the whole issue.

Where are these questions being asked? They come up everywhere—at work, at social events. At rituals that celebrate the turnings in life—weddings, baby showers. Even after funerals! But they are also being asked in ordinary, everyday sorts of get-togethers, in an atmosphere of conviviality and friendship. Well meaning. Interested. Not intending to hurt, not intending to pry.

And at one level a person knows this. And this just makes it worse, being reminded of what she, as well as everyone else, believes in.

> Another area that affects my identity that I don't feel comfortable with yet is this social pressure. Although I'm not that concerned—I'm more worried about me than what other people are thinking. But those karmas still throw me off. And I know that comments and questions aren't done maliciously—I don't know one person who would do it to hurt me. But they are awkward for me sometimes, and I

> wish . . . I feel like saying, 'It's hard enough—don't ask,' you know? And I'm not sure if it wasn't me, if I wouldn't be insensitive. I hope I would be sensitive—I never ask people if they are getting married because I got married late, too.
>
> —Theresa

Where did these attitudes come from? Attitudes that suggest childless persons are lesser people than those who are parents. Attitudes that suggest men and women aren't doing their job.

> I find that if you tell people who have children, or are expecting children, or just had children, they react to it very differently—almost like you have a disease. It's not like you have cancer or anything that drastic but there's something wrong with you. I think if we told this one couple, the wall would come up. They just had a baby. 'Oh, look, now she walks, now she talks, she smiles.' They'd worry about that because they would think it would upset us. And it doesn't. We can deal with it.
>
> —Carrie

If women and men start to pick apart these messages, trying to unravel why they feel bothered, they realize others' attitudes reflect their own unrealized expectations. Expectations that are embedded in the culture.

In our culture, it's parenthood, not marriage, that assigns us full status as adults, that says we are responsible citizens, that gives us equality with everyone else.

> People say to us, 'Oh, you can do anything you want, you don't have anything to tie you down.' And you're viewed as not as serious, eternally youthful, that you really don't have responsibilities. There's a lot of judgment. I'm sure you have heard this about people who don't have children. So we don't get taken quite as seriously as they do because they are a 'real' family.
>
> —Jenny

Women and men start to feel these values they believe in are loaded. Values become judgments, raining down on their heads. The hardest ones to hear are the intimations that childless couples are not adults yet because they don't have kids.

> I think it's partly the way other people treat you. You know, especially older women in middle age who have grown children and who are just beginning to have grandchildren. It's like, 'Oh, you're just a little kid because you haven't had children yet of your own,' and 'When you grow up, then you'll have kids, right?'
>
> —Susan

Being childless appears to disqualify women and men from being knowledgeable about a whole period of life: childhood. Even though they were kids once, and even though most of them have been around children their whole lives, they don't have the right credentials. Nothing they say counts, because they aren't parents yet themselves.

Women are harder hit by these attitudes than men because of their pivotal role in perpetuating the family life cycle. They find themselves growing more sensitive with each passing day, as the barbs and thoughtless comments of others go straight to the vulnerable spot in their identity.

Women need to find a means of self-protection. They need to marshal their defenses. But they may feel off guard, defenseless. Because they are faced with an even more immediate difficulty—being left behind.

BEING LEFT BEHIND

> LARRY: A couple of friends had their kids pretty early, and I felt less pressure then because we were busy doing other things. But this summer we were at a party for a friend's birthday, and four out of nine women were pregnant. Two had just found out. And last week my brother and his wife had their third child. So I feel some pressure.

> SUSAN: Right now is a real hard time because a lot of our friends who are our age are having kids. I mean, just everybody is pregnant. It makes you feel like you're the only one. It's in the media. Last month two movie stars got pregnant—they all do. And everyone at work is pregnant. It's like you can't get away from it no matter where you turn.

Friends trigger each other's biological clock.

We go through life making friends with others our age. We start early—in nursery school or grade school—and our minds and bodies develop in tandem. As we get older, being exactly the same age isn't so important. But usually our friends—especially our close friends—are within a few years of our own age. Being part of an age group means we go through life in the same stages. Sometimes we experience turning points in life together—maybe we graduated from college together, or became roommates with our first jobs. Sometimes we are drawn to each other because of similarities in our past. And sometimes because of what we share now.

Friends expect to go through life with each other. Sharing goals and dreams. Talking about whether to have children. Friends anticipate the future together, extending the preparations at home into the social arena. Together they explore what having children will mean for them. As women. As men. Friends encourage each other. They inspire each other. If they are eager to have children, they fan each other's enthusiasm. If they have cold feet, they hold each other's hand.

> My friends all got pregnant, and I was left behind. They knew that I was trying to get pregnant, too. They got pregnant and I didn't.
>
> —Sandra

Women are much more affected than men when friendships become emotionally cluttered by pregnancies and babies. When everyone else is pregnant and she is not, the cloud hanging over a woman's head grows larger. Conversations with friends have become monologues from which she feels excluded. Everyone talks about babies.

> I have about three close women friends and all of them had children in one year. It was very painful. They knew how I felt and they gave me a lot of space to avoid contact with them if I needed to. For me, the hardest part was when they would tell me that they were pregnant. Not once they were visibly pregnant, or after they delivered, or even seeing their kids—it was their announcement that did it.
>
> Then my best friend got pregnant. I avoided her for about two weeks. She knew I was going to need some time. Then when I could sort of deal with it, I told her it was hard and she understood, but it was terrible. It was really bad.
>
> —Dierdre

A woman feels ignored while her pregnant friends compare their due dates and how it feels to be pregnant. She feels a certain condescension whenever she volunteers anything about pregnancy or childbirth. Because what does she know? She hasn't experienced it yet. Pretty soon she shuts up. She stops talking.

> People think because we don't have children, we know nothing about them. We are so stupid. We're uninformed. We can't say that they walk at fifteen months, or they walk in a year. 'What do you know? You don't have kids.'
>
> —Carrie

Men usually don't notice at first that their partners aren't having fun. They are still talking to each other with animation. They're not talking about babies or pregnancy symptoms. They're talking about whatever they have always talked about—sports, the stock market, the deal they cut, the fish they caught. Whatever it has always been still goes on, for them.

Not only that, when women and men were all childless together, the gap between their pursuits didn't seem so great. Mutual interests cut across gender. Conversations ranged far and wide, covering topics of interest to everyone. Not anymore.

> I was sitting there one day with these friends of ours who are pregnant. He had his hand on her stomach and was saying, 'Was that a little heady or a little footy?' He was making such a jerk out of himself, I egged him on. Then they wonder why I don't want to go over there. They are very into possessions. They had the room decorated five months before the baby arrived. Then you have to go in and turn on all the little mobiles, and they turn around.
>
> —Judy

Women's daily lives are more affected than men's in the transition to parenthood. So it shouldn't come as a surprise that when a pregnancy occurs—when a child is born—women withdraw from their broader interests in life to focus on motherhood. This *is* a major life transition. And it deserves a woman's full attention. But when it's happening to everyone else, and not happening to her, it's hard to handle.

Men often aren't aware that women feel left out and can't talk so easily to their friends—until women tell them. Men may be surprised. They may resent it, and feel they are being put on the spot.

> It's stupid to go over and pretend to enjoy yourself. But my husband thinks I'm being terrible. I just don't feel that way. I think they are being terrible. I would never dream of insisting to someone who wasn't getting pregnant that they come to my baby shower. So it has certainly changed our lives. Our friends have dropped off, and the relatives I can't stand.
>
> —Judy

Suddenly a couple's social life has changed. They're not part of a foursome at that little Italian restaurant anymore. Instead, they're asked if they want to come along to McDonald's, where the kids can make noise. If a couple does continue to be part of a foursome with another couple who now has a child, it may get awkward, especially if a man and his best friend are having a great time together, and his partner suddenly can't bear to be around the best friend's wife and baby.

> Our very good friends just had twins and I've been avoiding them at all costs. They are mortified that we haven't come over to see them and cuddle their kids. Finally, this friend shows up at Vern's work one day and says, 'Why can't you come over and share our happiness?' So Vern had to tell him.
>
> —Judy

Women realize they need to start making some changes. To start protecting themselves from all this pain. But thinking about it is easier than doing it. Declining to attend the baby shower of a distant cousin may not be so hard, but it's a different story when it's a best friend's.

A woman tries to avoid the pain, a pain that has by now spread out to engulf her partner, too. It usually takes some time for her to realize she has to act, not just react, that she needs to set some policies and take a stand. Up to now, she has gone on fielding social situations, using all the skills she has developed in human relationships to get through each new skirmish intact.

But pretty soon, she starts feeling numb. Numb with pain. And to her dismay, just when she thinks she has mastered going numb, she isn't numb anymore. She's on the edge of tears throughout every social event, feeling tense beforehand and often feeling depressed afterward. Socializing, whether it's with intimate friends and their new baby, or with a crowd of semi-strangers, has become a living hell.

And it has become hell for her partner, too. He may feel just as miserable. But even if he isn't, he can no longer avoid knowing what it's like for her. He may be the recipient of her anger, the focal point for her tension and negative feelings. And as mad as he may get about catching her flack, he ultimately identifies with her distress and takes some of it on himself.

TAKING CHARGE

A team approach is the best way to ride out this era of your lives. You can maximize your effectiveness and minimize the pain and the long-term dislocations to your social relationships by joining forces and working through each issue together. After all, we are talking about the friends each of you has, and all of the people you know jointly as a couple—your entire social world. The team approach is, unfortunately, not going to banish pain, but it will recede to a tolerable level *most* of the time. And you will become more effective in handling social situations when you work in concert with each other.

How can I predict this will happen? When we handle our social relationships alone under these circumstances, the pain we feel is really the pain of loneliness, the pain of feeling, as Marsha did, that we are the "only one in the world." If you take charge of your social life together, you will have company.

You will find that strategizing over this area of your lives will increase your intimacy with each other. Every social encounter—every occasion that comes up—will necessitate that you put your heads together to decide what to do about that particular event, no matter how big or small. You will eventually develop a repertoire for how to cope, and sooner or later you will find yourself automatically plugging in the right strategy at the right time, then taking turns managing it.

> You meet people at parties and they say, 'When are you guys going to have kids?' I *feel* like saying, 'Well, we're not. We're both infertile. You want to talk about it?' But what we have actually done is develop a variety of approaches, from acting carefree, saying things like, 'Who needs kids?' to outright lying. Only our closest friends know. It's not something you can easily discuss with other people. They don't always understand.
>
> —Jenny

Good things will come of this effort. You will feel supported by each other. And you will feel less isolated from each other, which, in turn, has a ripple effect: You will feel less isolated from everyone else, too. You will stop feeling as if you are the only one in the world. Or, if you still feel that way, it won't be so hard to bear. And in time, you will begin to see the light at the end of the tunnel. Life *will* become normal again, no matter how disconcerting it is now.

TELLING OTHERS

One of the first issues to address together is who to tell. What happens when the decision is made to tell? Sometimes it's hard to gauge what others' response will be.

> GEORGE: At some point we made a conscious decision to tell people we had a problem, on the theory that keeping it to ourselves wasn't doing us any good, and maybe we could get people's sympathy and understanding.
>
> PENNY: It was like sexually coming out of the closest.
>
> GEORGE: Yeah, it didn't work at all. It backfired. People just didn't understand it. We started getting all the advice: take a vacation, just relax, blah, blah, blah.
>
> PENNY: And then they started asking us the most impertinent questions. They were insensitive. They would phone me every month to find out if I was pregnant.

Penny and George had the right idea when they decided to tell others about their fertility problem. But their efforts backfired because of the way they went about it—they indiscriminately told everyone.

Secrets are not a good thing. But it is important to differentiate *secrecy* from *privacy*.

Secrets are hidden from view. They imply a stigma. If we have a secret, we may feel shameful about it. Family secrets are like this—the skeletons in our closet that we don't want others to know about. Most people have a few of these, with feelings of shame attached to them. It's only because they have been kept secret that shame has grown up around them. Family secrets often belong to someone else—they happened in some other generation, and there was covert agreement to keep the secret. Or they happened to us, and we didn't know how to handle what happened, except to keep it secret. So the shame that surrounded those topics grew. And then they became *big* secrets, and the investment in keeping them hidden increased even more.

Just as family secrets become shameful by keeping them secret, so does infertility. Keeping infertility secret makes it seem like a fault that should be hidden. But infertility is no one's fault. Secrecy loads infertility with shame, with stigma—unnecessarily.

Angie was determined to keep the fertility problems she and Rick shared a secret from everyone, but especially from her family—even from her sister who had been infertile. But this amount of secrecy only served to heighten her feelings of shame.

> Infertility is a shame, you are ashamed. It is such a secret thing. It is so damned. When we first went to Resolve, we were laughing as we were getting out of the car, and I said to Rick, 'After all our years in the sixties and the dope and all this stuff, this is the most underground thing we have ever done. It's coming up publicly. But interpersonally it is still underground.

Her shameful feelings were fed by family attitudes about fertility, especially those of her mother:

> How did she do it—get pregnant? That is why I can't share it with her. Because she makes comments all the time about all they had to do was wipe their hands on the same towel and they were pregnant. I feel like saying, 'Oh, is *that* how you get pregnant?' But I don't. I say nothing.

While secrecy has all these connotations of shame that, in turn, reinforce feelings of isolation, privacy means something different. Privacy is a human need. Something private is something not shared because it is no one else's business, not because it is shameful. No matter how gregarious or open we may be, we all need privacy in some areas of our life.

A child first learns the idea of privacy upon being toilet trained. As the child grows, the notion of privacy expands to include other areas of life, whether it is through a teenage diary or in confidences shared with a best friend.

In adulthood, we recognize our personal boundaries, and within those boundaries we define the amount of space we need for our self. As we define ourselves and our needs better, many areas of our life become private, especially from persons outside our family.

The degree of privacy necessary for well-being varies greatly from one person to the next. We all have a need to keep things to ourselves, not because they are shameful, but because they are intimately linked to our identity, to the essence of who we are.

When we choose to share this essence with another person—when we make love with our partner or have a heart-to-heart talk with our best friend—we give the gift of ourselves—of intimacy, of trust. We are exposing our self and allowing another person to get close. At this level of intimacy, we are highly selective, and with good reason. When we open ourselves to others and admit them into our private world, we do so with the expectation that they will be respectful of our vulnerability and sensitive to our needs. Sharing intimate thoughts and feelings with close friends under these circumstances can bring self-acceptance, which has the power to heal. So telling others can be a good thing. Feelings of shame may dissipate, if telling is met with acceptance and compassion.

Keeping in mind what privacy means to you and your partner, select whom you tell accordingly. Once someone else knows, infertility ceases to be a secret. It is no longer coated in shame. But it continues to be a private matter. At some level of identity, infertility will always be a private matter, even if the whole world ultimately knows.

Over time, the need for privacy surrounding infertility may

dwindle and become unimportant. When this happens, you will know that infertility has lost its power over you—its ability to make you feel bad about yourself. When you can talk about your infertility without flinching inside, you will have reached a new sense of self-acceptance. By then, infertility won't be a secret anymore. It won't even be very private, and you will see no need to make it so. This is a goal to work toward, but at your own pace. It takes time.

It is wise to start by being selective about whom to tell—whom to sit down and talk with about it. Choose people you think will understand.

> I think you choose some of them carefully. You don't talk to everyone about it. One couple that we are friends with—my boss and his wife—you really could not talk to her about it. She is one of those people who just doesn't view life that way.
>
> —Larry

> I am very selective about who I open up to about this. I feel like now I'm getting enough support, and I don't need to say to everyone I meet, 'Hi, I'm infertile.' My feeling is when you are not selective, if you give a person that kind of information about yourself, you don't know what they are going to do with it. I don't want my problem to be coffee-break conversation.
>
> —Theresa

When you do confide in your friends, be prepared for *their* uncertainty. Friends *are* concerned. But it may get awkward because they often don't know how to respond—when to bring it up, when to leave it alone.

> When we were out walking, Lynn said, 'I don't know whether to ask you whether you are pregnant or not. If I don't say anything I'm afraid you will think I'm ignoring you, and if I do say something I'm afraid I'll hurt your

feelings.' So people don't even know the etiquette of how to handle you.

Another time we were up in the country with some friends, and one couple had a three-and-a-half-year-old boy. And you know, at that age they are going through whining. And he was whining. So my other friend and I left the house and went for a walk at one point because he and his mom were working on whining. And she said to me, 'Maybe you're really lucky—look at what it's like.' And I said, 'There are a lot harder things to do than have a ten-minute talk with a kid about whining. And waiting month after month to get pregnant is one of them. I would trade a ten-minute talk about whining for this any day.' People try to say the right thing to you, and they just keep sticking their foot in their mouth.

—Jenny

There *is* no etiquette for talking about infertility. Like many other conditions that have stigma attached to them, the person who feels stigmatized must *create* the etiquette and set out ground rules for others to follow. Doing so gives the individual a sense of personal power that may ameliorate, in part, the effects of the stigma. People may say awkward or odd things. They may seem overly aloof, or they may seem too interested. It is important not to let your extrasensitive feelings run away with you. Try to listen carefully to their responses or to what they say when they initiate the subject. Notice their body language, their feelings. What is important is the underlying sense of caring that is expressed, as Lynn attempted to show to Jenny. Respond to that, and just be yourself. Remember, you chose this person, probably for some very good reasons.

You might try saying something like, "Talking about infertility is awkward. There aren't any rules. Sometimes I feel like talking about it, and sometimes I don't. I'll try to be honest about my feelings."

If you can say this, or something like it, to those you have chosen to talk with, you are really making progress. It means you're able to keep your infertility in perspective. But if you can't say things like this yet—or if you can't talk about it at all—don't feel bad. This is a goal to work toward. Don't put yourself down if you can't do it yet. Keeping infertility in perspective is one of the hardest things you could possibly do.

Sometimes the people we choose to tell are at a loss. They don't know what to say or do, so they say *something* in an effort to be positive or accepting, but it just isn't the right thing. And then we are offended.

> The thing I resent the most from my friends who have children is, 'Oh, you can't have children? Come over and enjoy our children.' Like it's a new TV set. It's not the same thing.
>
> —Judy

> The worst thing in the world is when people want to give me good-luck charms. I hit the roof when one of my dearest friends wanted to give me this bracelet with charms on it that a friend had given her and she had gotten pregnant. I didn't scream and I didn't yell, but I told her in kind of a rude way that that was the worst thing you can do to someone like me. 'Let me just educate you about how to treat people. If we are going to be friends, you need to know that. What is wrong with us has nothing to do with luck, and I don't need your good-luck charm because what is happening to me is not bad luck. We are having real problems and that is why we can't conceive, and no amount of turtles under my pillow or beads or tea is going to help.'
>
> —Cindy

> The thing I had a problem with were the smart-ass remarks: 'Well, your husband can't get you pregnant, let's go into the next room.' That kind of thing. Kenny got that kind of thing, too. When I heard remarks toward him, 'What is wrong with you?' that hurt me more than the kind of stuff that I got because I felt I was able to handle it.
>
> —Dorene

Sometimes a couple gets the message, "Try harder." This is part of our cultural heritage, our national ethic—the Horatio Alger story applied to infertility:

> The worst is when people think—my friend John is one example of it, and my mother believes it a little bit, too—that if you try hard enough, you will get pregnant. We get this all the time. In the last State of the Union Message, the gist was, 'Try harder.' When the President is saying, 'Anybody in this country can make it if they only try hard enough,' you realize it's our national ethic. So, I guess, what else should we expect them to believe?
>
> —Larry

Talking to others about infertility isn't easy, although it does get easier with time. And often women and men don't get the response they want or the support they need. Consequently, women, who get the brunt of questions, work at figuring out better ways to deal with the subject.

> I was watching Dolly Parton in an interview on TV. Someone mentioned something about kids, and she says, 'I can't have kids.' It was really neat to see her sort of spit it out, there was no fumbling, it was just the way it was. So it has given me an incentive. I have to practice doing that.
>
> —Belinda

Penny and Susan both reflected on their strategies, ones that you can perhaps amend to work for you:

> With many people I have learned I can deal with it simply by changing the course of the conversation without being direct. I find that they cannot deal with me saying I don't want to talk about it. Then they wonder what is the matter and ask, 'Why are you upset?' So if I can turn the subject to themselves, which is their favorite subject anyway, I do. That works.
>
> —Penny

> I haven't yet figured out a technique for answering the question, 'Do you have any children?' that is a clear message that says, 'This is the end of the discussion.' I can't bring myself to say, 'No, and no more is going to be said or asked about it. It would be very rude to pursue this line of questioning.' I haven't figured out how to do that yet. It's going to take some practice. Just by giving out that much, it opens it up for discussion. Maybe just a simple *no* is the best thing to say. 'No, we don't.' Period.
>
> —Susan

Sometimes, in spite of all efforts, friendships are lost. Usually, these are friendships between women. The relationship brings up too much grief, too much anger, too much pain, to keep it going.

> One of the first friends I made here, she became pregnant three months later, after I miscarried, and she was very self-involved. Which was appropriate. That was okay. But we couldn't maintain the friendship. It was too difficult to do.
>
> —Belinda

> What I did was I withdrew from one person. I just couldn't be around that child without feeling really sad. And it's still there when I talk about it, when I remember the sadness and how hard it was for me to watch all my friends get pregnant.
>
> —Sandra

A couple starts rethinking the whole script they made for themselves. What if it doesn't turn out the way they planned it?

> CARRIE: If we don't have children, it will be a void because we'll always be an enigma. Most people our age are married with several kids. So most of our friends have become single people because our activities are geared that way. Yet we are a couple. So we're always going to have a problem in that regard.

> RUSS: Yeah. We don't know where we fit in.
>
> CARRIE: We don't fit in now, actually. Because most of the people who don't have children are having them now. And that's hard.

Women and men spend more and more time with their still-childless friends. If they have any friends who aren't planning to have children, it's a relief. Because children don't come up in the conversation. It's a reminder there's a whole life out there without children.

> SUSAN: I guess in some ways you kind of cling to those people who don't have children. Because you feel like at least they won't reject you if you don't have children. Even though a lot of them are kind of starting to change their minds. We have one set of friends who have decided they definitely do not want to have children. And even they are rethinking that.
>
> LARRY: I don't think so. I asked them again. And they said, 'No,' so I think they are a potential source of support.

When women and men socialize with single friends, they don't have to anticipate each encounter, wondering how they will respond this time to volleys of, "When are you two going to have children?" They can just relax.

> Our single friends—it's sort of beyond their ability to understand. They don't worry about it. Their response is, 'Oh, no success getting pregnant? Well, good—we can go out and party!' That's the way they look at it—that we're available, we're not tied down.
>
> —Carrie

The answer doesn't lie in just sticking with single friends, though. Women and men don't want to miss out on their other relationships. The friends who are preoccupied with becoming parents now are important. Otherwise, so much energy wouldn't have been plowed into building friendships with them in the first place. It's hard work building a friendship. When a friendship fades because of infertility, it's a loss, *another* loss, one we can ill afford at this time in life. It's important to find ways to keep these relationships and enjoy them.

Friends are only one issue. The other big issue looms just as large. What to do about family?

CHAPTER 7

FAMILY MATTERS

Whatever kind of family we come from, when we find a partner, we bring our families with us. They may be central in our life. Or they may be peripheral. Family members may be more than family—they may be our friends, too. Maybe our family is not so important for the role they play in our life now—it's their presence in our past and what that means for the future that matters. Regardless of how often we see them or how close we are, we feel their presence in other ways—through the powerful emotional bond that links us to them. A bond that is infinitely complex.

As women and men prepare to re-create the family, they want to perpetuate this bond between their families and the next generation. It's an American value to be a close-knit family. We were all raised on stories of three- and four-generation families. No matter what our race or creed, this is the story of "it used to be."

Why is family so important? Good parent-child relations are a cultural expectation. As a couple starts the next generation, they want to renew and strengthen their ties with the generation that came before. It's an assumption everyone makes about generational continuity, that it's the task of soon-to-be parents to nurture this bond. To connect the past with the future. There is social pressure to do this, to be the connecting link.

> I only have one brother, and he's not married, so if they are going to have grandkids, I'm the one who is going to produce them. But I think the pressure for that is probably more internal from me than it is from them. I would like to.

> Part of having a grandchild is that I know it would make them really happy.
>
> —Susan

Each family is unique. Nevertheless, some of the qualities in a woman's family are usually mirrored in her partner's family. Or their families may seem like opposites, reflecting their own distinctive personalities. Some of these qualities inevitably spill over into the relationship. The family issues that arise when a couple is trying to conceive are an amalgam of this process. It's their family soup, thick with history and loaded with the ingredients for both peace and conflict. If they can identify the contents—what gives it flavor, what stirs it up, and when to serve it—they may be able to develop a workable plan for this time in their lives. Gina and Greg were forced to deal with a variety of family issues as they struggled with their infertility.

> GINA: My father is one of those people who is never, ever going to give approval for who you are and what you stand for. I've written him off on a lot of levels. I would very much like to have his approval but I'm not going to get it. We found out as of last year that he was having trouble forgiving Greg and me for living together before we were married. Now that was ten years ago, mind you. We have been happily married for eight. So he is not quite in this world.
>
> GREG: And my mom. . . . Basically, my mom is a practicing grandmother without a license. In the absence of her children providing her with grandchildren, she has moved on to adopting nieces and nephews. We have a very prolific wing of the family, and they have, I don't know—five hundred nieces and nephews—there is quite a number of the little brats running around. And so she has adopted them. The stories of what she bought for Christmas and Easter, and they came over and did this and that. All the chitter-chatter about children got to be too much for us.
>
> So we took some very deliberate steps. We would never

just sit down and talk about it. Both of us come from families that are nonconfrontational about medical and sexual problems. So it wasn't an encounter group experience with our families. We didn't have the resources to say, 'Hey, let's sit down and have a heart-to-heart talk.'

Men and women will probably renegotiate the course of action they want to take with their families many times along the way, as Greg and Gina did:

GREG: We found an article for parents and friends of infertile couples, a Resolve publication.* We gave that to both sides of the family and they acknowledged that they got it and understood. Now both sides of the family basically are obvious by their exclusion of the topic. So it is louder than a whisper would be. Well, actually, for a while they laid off, but now they are getting back.

GINA: It's nearly impossible to make someone else understand the pain. Especially the stupid little comments, the constant barrage that you deal with and the constant goddamn grandkid pictures, and all that stuff. They have to be reminded now and then. When I get pumped about my sister's children, 'What are they doing?' I have to say, 'I don't like to talk about that, thank you.' Well, why not? 'Well, in ten words or less . . .' and you sort of have to rehit them on the head again.

They care a great deal, they just . . . Greg's family didn't talk about that kind of thing. They don't know what to say.

*Resolve has a publication for family members that is available from their national headquarters.

TALKING WITH PARENTS

When you and your partner consider talking with your parents, it helps if you ask yourselves some basic questions: What do our families know? Do we let them in on what is going on? What do we tell them? Do we tell them anything? What if they keep bringing up grandchildren? Do we talk about it? *Can* we talk about it? Or do we clam up? Do we want them to be in the dark? Why?

Angie didn't want her family to know, and she had a specific reason:

> I don't want my family to know. Until you're involved with it you don't know what it means. He's not sterile, but he has a low sperm count. What does that mean? All they hear is sperm count, low sperm count. They know nothing. My mother and father conceived three children and didn't think about it. I have a cousin who has an infertility problem. And my mother knows about him, and she gets off on it. A man who has a problem is suspect.

Although Angie had a specific reason for not talking with her family, many women and men are less clear about their hesitancy. Do we choose what we do in relation to our families? Or is it a matter of instinct? There are no right answers to these questions. Everyone has reasons for following a certain path. But sometimes it helps to stop and ask yourself what those reasons are in order to prepare for the next step.

> My mother wouldn't expect me to discuss our problem with her. The way I was raised, something like infertility is a subject for discussion between me and my husband only. She is careful not to intrude on our relationship.
>
> —Paula

> I've always wanted to have kids. My mom told me when I was young—she always used to tease me and say, 'If you ever get pregnant, we will keep the baby.' So she already wanted a grandkid. When I was about 16 she said, 'If you get pregnant, we will keep it, you don't have to give it up. You don't have to have an abortion.' So I told her—I knew she would see me through this, too.
>
> —Donna

> She has still done more than me—she has had kids. I don't want to get into it with her. I wouldn't give her the satisfaction of letting her know I was having trouble getting pregnant. She didn't treat me like an adult until I got married. If I told her about the infertility, I would lose my equality.
>
> —Laura

And what about your in-laws? You may feel distant from them, or you may have adopted them. Either way, you didn't grow up in that family, so communication may be uncertain around complicated issues. No matter what approach you decide to take, you and your partner should work on this together. In-law jokes are alive and well. They don't need more fuel. You and your partner may ask yourselves, "Should we present a united front? Or is this a solo endeavor?" The answer probably depends on the nature of your family relationships.

> Russ's mother was awful. She thinks, and whatever she thinks just comes out of her mouth. She doesn't think hard enough about what she says. Because we are having no luck, her tactic was to say, 'Well, one of the happiest couples I know doesn't have children.' Well, that's fine but we want children. Please don't use that as any solace or condolence.
>
> So we kept hearing this, and finally I said, 'Russ, if your mom says that one more time . . .' So Russ jumped on her. He got his mother all upset. She does have five kids so I can understand her not being that worried about us

having kids. And she didn't have any help, so it was a handful.

—Carrie

When you and your partner consider telling parents you are trying, ask yourselves if your parents will understand. You are probably wondering if, by telling parents, you will get what you need from them. Ask yourselves, "Are they on our wavelength? Will they be able to listen? Will they be able to understand what it is like? After all, they succeeded where we have not—they had us. Will they accept us on our terms? Will we get support? The kind of support we want?" Susan and Larry asked themselves these questions before they approached their families.

SUSAN: My mother didn't get married until she was 32. So she didn't even start her family until then. And she wasn't real sure she would be able to have kids. She had several miscarriages in the beginning. So I think that probably makes somewhat of a difference; they were both older. I think they came to the whole thing with a different perspective.

LARRY: It's very difficult for my mother to be supportive. She's not the kind of person you think of as a really supportive person because she's really got her own twitch. But at the same time, when she can make the time, she is really wonderfully solicitous. I think she really, truly does care about us and wants us to be happy. And is one of life's great, incurable optimists. But you can't talk sense to her.

SUSAN: Yeah, but she's been real supportive.

LARRY: Yeah. So she's actually been pretty good about it, I think. And my father—my parents got divorced some years ago, and my father got remarried. I would say that he is basically oblivious to things he is not into.

Getting Needs Met

When Susan and Larry told their parents about the problems they were having conceiving, they were fairly sure they would get some of what they needed. Most couples who think they will get *some* of what they need usually tell their families. They need support, and they will take whatever they can get. Belinda was no exception:

> I probably tell her more about the problems I am having than she wants to hear, not that she doesn't care, but she just doesn't know how to deal with it. My gut feeling is that she feels bad about it. But maybe that is just wishful thinking. But when she came to visit, she helped with the adoption letters. So she can't really express it verbally but she can do things, and that is kind of her way. I know she cares about me and about us, and loves us, but it is just kind of where she is at.

Sometimes men and women anticipate they will not get support, and the telling would simply make more work. When parents appear oblivious, their child thinks twice about telling them, as Jenny did:

> My mother is off in her own world, taking care of my father, traveling, socializing with her friends. I think she thinks it would make her old.

A couple may decide to avoid the whole topic, if they think their families have already come to their own conclusions.

> LAURA: My family doesn't mention having children and Stan's family doesn't mention it. I think they think we're too old.

> STAN: I think my folks are cool. They both realize we are over 40, and they are not giving us any static at all. They probably don't expect any grandchildren. I think they figure we are beyond the age in life.

When a couple does tell their parents, sometimes it works out fine. They get what they need, and, as time passes, they usually continue to get their needs met, as Susan did:

> I think my parents have really been there for us, overall. Last time—I don't know about my mother—she said something about how 'you really can have a great life without kids, too.' And she's reinforcing that. That makes me feel good.

If that's the case, it's not an issue. End of subject.

For many women and men, though, that's not the end of the subject because parents have all kinds of attitudes and feelings about this. It's the future of *their* family, too, as Laurel was reminded.

> In Earl's family, there are four kids. He is the only one without kids. For a long time his father kept asking when we would have kids. We never said anything. Earl would just joke and say, 'We don't know how.' So they wrote up their will, and it was like people with kids were getting more.

And it has become a sensitive topic. Laurel felt slighted:

> That bothered me. They are so children-oriented. I know kids are cute, but we are people, too.

Sometimes everybody gets into the act. Men and women may have a lot of trepidation about what will happen if their infertility becomes public property. This is always a possibility. Donna explained what happened when she and Ned "went public":

> One of the bad things is you tell everybody—well, that is good because you have to get it out there. But the bad part

> about it is after that everybody, every month, asks if anything happened. And it never does, and that's real hard. The people closest to me quit doing it—my mom quit doing it, my stepsister. I finally asked my stepsister to shut up about anything to do with it. She would do it in front of the whole family at Christmas and Thanksgiving. In front of everybody in my family. And I would have to smile and say, 'Well, we are working on it.' And try to make jokes and stuff.

If it's a woman's in-laws, ultrasensitive feelings may be involved. She wants equal time and attention with her sisters- and brothers-in-law. And she is angry if she feels she's not getting it—if she feels left out.

> I talk to my mother-in-law, and sometimes she's supportive. But I have noticed that there's a real difference in her attitude toward me and toward my sister-in-law who has the same problem. With her, it's a real tragedy.
>
> —Jenny

So she is often jealous:

> I'm bound and determined not to go down and see my brother-in-law's family until their baby is walking and talking and has its own personality. It has caused a lot of problems. After Vern's father died, I used to go down and cook his family Thanksgiving dinner. I just flat out refused to do it this year. I said, 'If you want to go, go, and I'll take care of myself.' I don't know. Men don't get those jealousies. Women do.
>
> —Judy

MOTHERS AND DAUGHTERS

Talking with parents usually means a daughter talking with her mother. Fathers don't usually enter into it much. The information gets relayed to Dad by his wife:

> My father and I don't usually talk on that level. We have talked some on that level, but not as much. There is just a different relationship there.
>
> —Sheila

The same is true for sons, who usually tell their mothers. But sometimes, depending on how close partners feel to their in-laws, they may talk with their parents together.

> We told Hal's parents, and they were real upbeat. They live out in the country, 'Everything's okay, you're okay.' My family were doomsayers. Everything bad was going to happen. They were the opposite ends of the spectrum.
>
> —Marsha

If parents are divorced, a father may not even know.

> I haven't seen my father since . . . well, he is in the process of moving across the country. I told my younger brother who lives down south. But I haven't heard from my father yet. My mom lives across the freeway.
>
> —Dennis

If fathers do get into the act, it's usually because they have some specific knowledge to be tapped:

> My father is a GP. He was reassuring. He has seen a lot of women with problems who later had children.
>
> —Al

Sometimes this expertise is a mixed blessing.

RUSS: My father is a retired doctor and my uncle is a doctor. Neither of them knows about this field but they get into the act a lot. My father has had some impact on our state of mind. They both have opinions about what is being done and whether it is appropriate.

CARRIE: That was too much. In fact, I was quite irritated by it. I got tired of having three doctors—four doctors actually, if you count your uncle, telling me what we should do and writing up my history. Your father is so blunt I felt like it was an invasion of my privacy, some of the things that he wrote.

RUSS: Yes, but I appreciated their good intentions.

Relationships between mothers and daughters are complicated at the best of times. But a woman's experience is different from her mother's when she is having no success with conception. This difference may potentially strain communication. Yet this is a time of life when a woman wants to feel especially close to her mother.

A woman needs her mother now. For many reasons.

A woman wants that feeling of unconditional love—of being loved for herself as she is. She especially needs it right now. She wants her mother to undo those bad feelings she has about herself. Because her mother is in a position to ease the pain better than anyone else. If the woman who mothered her and raised her to follow in her maternal footsteps—if she can say the right words of comfort—it will cushion her daughter from some of her pain. She can make it okay—well, more okay than anybody else can. She has the power to reduce her daughter's misery. She can take the sting out of the attitudes that plague her child because of who she is and what she stands for.

She can do this in many ways. By acknowledging her daughter's pain. By defusing her sense of failure. By reaffirming her daughter's identity as a woman and as a person of worth. And knowing her child so well, she will instinctively know what to say. And how to say it, as four different women attest:

> My mom is really distressed that I haven't been able to have children. I mean, my *mom* . . . She *knows* . . . I grew up wanting a child.
>
> —Sally

> My mother and I can talk on a really deep emotional level.
>
> —Sheila

> My mother basically has no comment other than, 'Well, do keep trying.' My mother is not the type to go into a long dissertation on the subject. For which I am very grateful.
>
> —Carrie

> My mom has just been great, which has been great for me.
>
> —Celia

Is this always realistic, this expectation? Is this a human-size task? Or an expectation for a larger-than-life mother? Maybe she can't do it. Maybe women are expecting too much.

If a parent has taken on the mother role with her whole being, she may not be able to do it. She will be paralyzed by her daughter's plight. She will understand the enormity of what her child is experiencing. She will be tongue-tied, guilt-stricken. Belinda described her painful efforts to talk with her mother:

> Since I'm having problems, I have asked her a number of times, 'Mom, does it bother you that you took DES and now we have these problems?' My mom's pat answer to everything is, 'Oh, not at all!' I don't know if it does or it doesn't, it appears to be denial. It's like, 'I don't want to talk about it.'

She will wonder about *herself*. How does this reflect on *her*, the mother? She may not be able to get outside of herself, as Dierdre unhappily learned:

> My mother had endometriosis before I was born.* One of the family stories has always been, 'I almost divorced your father because I thought I couldn't give him children.' Italian man, he would need children. Of course, she got pregnant with me and then she had three others. She was 22 when I was born.
>
> So when I had surgery, I called her and asked her to come because I wanted my mom. So she came with me and Terry to the hospital. When they unexpectedly took out my ovary, they went for coffee. My mother's a little dingy. Terry was blown away at that point that they took it out. He was talking with her. My mother ended up crying for herself, instead of supporting him. It reactivated her, her own issues around it. She cried in the coffee shop because of what happened to her. It was real interesting. She was very scared that she was never going to get pregnant. It sort of reactivated that memory.
>
> Since then, I don't know. I was very close to my mother when I was a kid, but now that I am an adult, I get really pissed with her. I see things a lot differently. I'm very angry with her. I think part of it is that motherhood has been her bailiwick and being a professional has been mine. I've always been pretty sad about it.

Most of all, she won't be able to live her daughter's experience with her. And that is what her daughter needs. Theresa analyzed her feelings after talking to her mother:

> My mother—I love my mother—but it's not working. She doesn't talk to me about it, ever. She has said it's not her strength. I don't get a good feeling, a good support feeling. I figured it is just her, she's not comfortable with it. But I'm not sorry I told her.

---

*Endometriosis is caused by the growth of endometrial cells outside the uterus—most typically in the ovaries and tubes, the abdomen, or the exterior of the uterus.

> I asked her if she had taken DES, and her comment was, 'No, I didn't, why would I have needed that?' It was like, if I had been real sensitive, I would have been hurt by the comment. It wasn't real tactful. It was sort of—'They gave it to people who had trouble, and that wasn't a problem for me.' Because she had six children.

If a woman was a reluctant mother—if she felt inadequate to the task, if she was resentful about the loss of a career, if she felt overloaded with babies, or felt they came too soon—she still won't be able to do it. Because now she is making up for lost time. She may make light of her daughter's struggle, without meaning to. If she had plans for her daughter that included making a mark on the world because she herself did not, she may be ambivalent. Or she may be conflicted, remembering the times she wished she had stayed single longer, the times she wanted to drop the burden of care and go off and play. Sometimes she did. Some daughters live with that, as Sarah does:

> Even to this day, my siblings say they look to me as the mother, and not to our real mother. Because our mother was this dreamy kind of person who was just trapped in this role. And didn't want to be in it. She was a little on the flaky side and not real nourishing. So I took over the mother role. If they have a problem, they call me.

If this was motherhood for a woman's mother, that mother may feel as inadequate to the task now as she did then. Helpless to help. She will hear her daughter's frustration with infertility. But she will not be able to identify with it. Because part of her will think, "Why? This is your chance to escape."

It's not surprising that so many mothers don't fit the cultural script for being the mom-that-meets-all-needs. It's a script for Superwoman, not for an ordinary mortal. Probably few mothers can measure up completely.

If a woman's mother doesn't fit the image of the perfect mother, she probably knew it already. But she doesn't want to be reminded. Not now. She wants the cultural script. The right words. Whatever they are. She wants comfort. Jenny was no exception.

> JENNY: So then we talked to my mother about it.
>
> MATT: Your mother is useless.
>
> JENNY: Yeah, my mother is really sort of flaky. Her idea of being a supportive grandmother would be to have booties delivered from I. Magnin to the front door.

No matter what, the culture reinforces a woman's hopes for her mother's ability to spread balm on her wounds. Reminding a woman that she and her mother should be close. Saying that mothers and daughters have a unique bond. So if things aren't perfect, a daughter feels cheated. And she feels like a failure, too. As a daughter. And as an aspiring mother.

> She believes that because she is my mother, she has a right to know everything. And because she is my mother, I have a very difficult time dealing with her. The only way I have learned to be able to do that with this subject is simply to lie.
>
> —Penny

> Frankly, I don't think my mom deals with this DES thing very well. I can't blame her. It's horrible. It's a very difficult situation. There are no days when I can sit down and talk about it with my mother. I don't know what I want from her. Do I want her to cry and plead and say, 'I'm sorry,' which she has already done at least once or twice? What good is that? There is not a whole lot either one of us can do about it, other than feel miserable about it. So I try to not inflict it upon her. I find talking with her about it extremely difficult.
>
> —Gina

There's no room in our mythology about mothers for variations on the Mom myth. So a woman may feel a huge loss if her story doesn't fit the cultural script. In real life, there are so many variations. What if a woman didn't have a mother growing up? That was Judy's experience.

> My mother died when I was 4. I was a latchkey child. I've always wanted my own family. I think, partially, it's never having known my own mother. It's somehow a way of resolving that relationship. It's like, not only am I going to be a mother, I'm going to have been somebody's daughter, too. It's a very strange kind of desire. I think it is a little bit different from the mothering instinct.
>
> I think a lot of it has to do with not knowing my own mother. I'm very curious as to what that relationship would have been, and I used to fantasize—'well, maybe she didn't die, maybe she ran away, maybe she couldn't stand my dad, she is really living somewhere.' And if I found out where, I would get on a plane and go find her. I never found out exactly what she died from. So I want an answer to this because I never had an answer to that.

What if a woman has lost her mother as an adult, like Laurel did?

> I feel like I'm missing out on a lot. Before she died, I said to my mom, 'I'm really sorry you didn't see us get married. Or have kids.' She said it didn't matter. For a long time I thought I didn't want children if she couldn't be there to share. So that was foremost in my mind after she died. I wouldn't be able to call her up. She wouldn't be there for Christmas. That really hurt. Then later I thought maybe it would be good to have a child because that would be part of her. So I started thinking about that. Earl thinks if we have a little girl, we should name her after my mom. Her death did influence me, first negatively, but later positively.

If a woman mothered her own mother, then she is still on the giving end. Instead of getting support, a daughter has to support her mother. Something is screwy about this. A daughter is doing all this extra work, and yet she still feels like a failure as a daughter. Dierdre was caught in this bind:

> I'm giving my sister a baby shower tomorrow. She's due. It's really interesting to watch how my mom deals with her pregnancy. It's not something she actively pursues being excited about. I had to really twist her arm to get her to come tomorrow. 'Oh, I have to work, I have to work.' 'Mom, come to the shower; Kitty is only going to have one baby the first time. You should be there.' 'You think so?' 'Yes.' Okay, then she comes.
>
> I don't know. I'm sure there are a lot of psychological issues involved with it. You can go crazy thinking it is all in your mind. It isn't all in my mind. There are issues that overlap. She wanted me to reassure *her*. Those are our roles. I take care of her that way. She worries, and I say, 'Mom, it's all right.'

So if a woman tells her mother what's happening, she may add a new, sometimes impossible burden to her ever-growing load: the feat of making it all right. This is what happened to Marsha.

> My mother's reaction—my mother is a whole other issue because she has enough guilt without being a DES mother to fuel an army. In general. She's not a happy woman at all. I told her what the doctor had said. I think, in part, I wanted sympathy, but I told her that she couldn't blame herself because in 1949 to tell a doctor that you didn't want to take DES was like saying you didn't want to take penicillin when you had pneumonia. They would have locked her up. She had had four miscarriages before me. They were documented. Apparently that doesn't make it better for my mother, because here she is responsible for my unhappiness. So that was a big deal. There was a general crisis.

Women emotionally load this scenario through their plans—plans to follow in their mother's footsteps. A woman wants that heightened sense of closeness, that bond, that so-important connection between herself and her mother. To not get it at this time of life creates an additional sense of loss.

Once a woman begins to think about what it is like to have a child, she feels wonder when she thinks about that long-ago event. Her own birth. When she was nurtured through her mother's umbilicus. When she was born. That she survived. This *is* a miracle—conception and birth. In preparing to have children, Sheila relived her own birth.

> My mother had a stillborn before me. She had an extremely difficult time having me. I was four pounds, four ounces at birth. I was a month in the hospital and I almost didn't make it. And it was very rough. The doctor told her no more children. He said, 'You are never to have any more children because it is too risky, not only for the baby, but for your life.' My mom was in there a long time, and my dad was driving back and forth. So she knows what it's like.

Enveloped by her feelings, Sheila felt moved in her mother's presence.

> My mother just had surgery for cancer. And that really hit me. I am very, very close to my mother. And I just thought, 'Why now, God?' I could give up my mother because I've had her for all these years of wonderful memories. But I'm selfish enough to want that for my children.
>
> And as much as I want a baby—I told my mom this—'I would rather give up a newborn baby than you. I can't have another mother. I can't establish that relationship with another woman.'

A woman's mother is a symbol. Of Womanhood. Of Motherhood. No matter how she did it, she bore a child. She raised a daughter. A woman doesn't realize what the task entails. Until now. Now that she is going to repeat the experience. Now that she has been trying to navigate the first step, she appreciates how difficult the whole process can be. She may feel inadequate to the task.

CHAPTER 8

FEELINGS

Not getting what we want when we want it stirs up a lot of feelings. Even if we finally get what we want but not according to plan, it's hard to take. We feel a sense of loss. And we feel angry because we feel we have been cheated, that somehow we have been robbed of the full promise of our lives. We feel anguish, pain. It's an ache that doesn't dissipate, that grows as time passes. It brings up old pain.

> I remember when I was little, and Janie sold me her doll. A half hour later her mother called to say she couldn't sell her toys. I had to give this doll back! The memory I have is my mother is seven months pregnant, and I am crying to beat the band on my mother's stomach as they take the doll away. Everybody else has a doll, how come I don't? It was very, very sad. It was hard. Infertility has that same kind of meaning for me.
>
> —Dierdre

Infertility is a metaphor for life's struggles. It comes at a time when women and men are dealing with the issues of mid-life—of letting go of impossible expectations and acknowledging loss. Of finding inner strength and self-acceptance. Of growing and changing. Of knowing oneself more fully. Of becoming one's true self, and moving toward the next stage of life.

Infertility precipitates grief for something that has not come to pass—the perfect pregnancy and the easily attained child. The loss women and men associate with infertility is intangible. This intangible quality makes infertility difficult to acknowledge and harder still to mourn.

> I've done more crying in the last year. It is hard to handle. Someone said it is grieving over the death of someone you have never known. And you don't have any prescribed roles—ways to handle it or respond to it.
>
> —Susan

We grieve for our losses at every stage of life. No matter what the loss entails—whether it is the loss of a person, a relationship, a role—even the loss of our dreams, we must mourn the loss in order to let go. We do this starting in childhood. The "terrible twos," for example, are about mourning—mourning the loss of the symbiosis of parent and child. But even while throwing a temper tantrum in the supermarket, the small child is not only grieving but letting go as well. As we grow up and grow older, we become more aware of the losses we face. We may first understand loss when we put away the toys of childhood, or when a much-loved grandparent dies. We anticipate some of our losses, while others are completely unexpected.

Infertility is an unexpected loss. The imagined child is not replaceable, no matter what comes later—pregnancy and childbirth, adoption, being childless. When infertility doesn't go away—with an easy pregnancy or a change of heart—then it has to be mourned. Women and men grieve so they can let go of their dream of the perfect child, their illusions of the perfect life.

> It's the idea of a baby. No one knows more about being pregnant, labor, and delivery than I do. I want people to tell me their labor and delivery stories of childbirth in minute detail. I have always been that way.
>
> —Marsha

This is why infertility lingers, even when it has become part of the past. Grieving is essential because it enables women and men to live with the loss infertility represents and go on to the next phase of life.

There are no rites of passage or other rituals to mark infertility as important in a person's life, even though it is a life event akin to birth, marriage, and death. It is hidden from view, a secret grief that is sometimes misunderstood by others when it is known.

Throughout the world, formalized rituals acknowledge and carry people through life events. When there is no such opportunity for the expression of emotions, all of the usual social avenues through which life events are legitimized are blocked. The individual is left with the full burden for navigating the transition rather than sharing it with others through society's usual channels. The hidden nature of infertility precludes public mourning or support—mechanisms that work to solidify bonds between people and carry them through times of hardship.

> Infertility is just such a strange thing. The difference between it and any other crisis is that you cannot share it publicly. Any other crisis you get sympathy for—it is ritualistic, it's acknowledged. That is an important thing—to be acknowledged. I wonder if infertility is acknowledged in other cultures.
>
> —Angie

Women go through a series of stages as they grieve, stages that are fraught with different emotions. These feelings are intense, as women grieve over the erosion of their control over their body.

> I feel more on an even keel now. I have been on this roller coaster for the last year, but now I feel better. Christmas was fine, the next month was fine. And then it sort of dipped again. I feel stronger now. It has been a roller coaster for me. I don't know what to attribute it to—events that cause it, or hormones, or what.
>
> —Theresa

Angie grappled with the abstract nature of the loss in her efforts to come to terms with it:

> In some ways infertility is incomparable to anything else because until you resolve it, you go through different stages.

> And on top of that, every month you get your period and start over again. It is just such an odd thing to live with.

DENIAL

After the discovery of infertility, women may continue for a long time to expect their infertility to be solved and conception to occur—sometimes for years on end.* Medical treatment and the reproductive cycle conspire to foster denial, as each new cycle brings new hope. Always looking ahead to the next cycle may perpetuate a sense of hopefulness that only begins to wane after the passage of time:

> I think denial played a big part in it, because we kept hoping. As time went on, our hope sort of dwindled because nothing came through.
>
> —Dierdre

> It's just an insane hope and there is no reason. Every month you hope that this month one sperm will find that one egg.
>
> —Molly

Denial enables women and men to deal with an intolerable situation in stages. It may initially serve a useful function, as women prepare themselves gradually to face the possibility that they may not have a genetic child. The enormity of the loss is too great to be taken in all at once. Women, especially, filter reality so that they can gradually face their infertility. This filtering process reduces the impact of infertility on a woman's identity so that she is able to go on functioning in her daily life. Gradual adjustment to the possibility that she may not bear a biological

*Approximately half of all persons who are diagnosed as infertile eventually have a biological child. As time passes without a conception, however, the likelihood of conception recedes and is a clue that other options should be explored.

child enables a woman to amend her sense of self-consistency over time.

> I am thinking that subconsciously there was a long period of preparation for what has happened, that somewhere down deep there was the thought, 'I won't have children,' or 'I'm infertile,' or something like that.
>
> —Theresa

Although denial may serve a protective function in earlier stages of infertility, as time goes by it may compound the pain and retard the process of resolution. When years pass, denial keeps women in bondage to their infertility. When Lisa became pregnant, she could not face the possibility that there might be a problem:

> When I finally got pregnant, my doctor decided I should have a sonogram. And they couldn't find anything in the uterus on the sonogram. He didn't look on that as very favorable, but I couldn't see it. I just thought there was something wrong with the sonogram, that they weren't able to read it. I was really denying that something was wrong. I finally agreed on a laparoscopy to see if it was an ectopic. I went into it thinking everything would be all right, that the sonogram would be wrong. He found a tubal pregnancy. I remember waking up in the recovery room and they were asking if I wanted a private or a shared room. I knew right then they had done a lot more than a laparoscopy, that I wasn't pregnant anymore.*

The magnitude of the loss was too difficult for Lisa to face. She reassured herself the way that many women do:

---

*A sonogram is a noninvasive procedure that takes a picture of a woman's tubes and uterus. A laparoscopy, diagnostic surgery to look at the condition of a woman's tubes, is minor surgery, and a woman is usually discharged from the hospital the same day. An ectopic pregnancy is a pregnancy that occurs in a tube instead of in the uterus, and must be terminated in major abdominal surgery.

> I don't really think I grieved. I am not really sure how I handled it. I just pulled myself back together and hoped that my chances would be good again because I had been able to get pregnant.

After ten years of infertility Lisa was still denying the unlikelihood of a successful pregnancy:

> It's still too soon to quit. Because I'm still ovulating and I still have a chance. Only now I have a lot more to weigh. My husband is at the end of his rope. He really can't tolerate much more. So now it's not just figuring out what I do next, but what he can handle, too.

Men also attempt to deal with infertility through denial. In other chapters I describe the different pace at which partners acknowledge a problem. The slowness with which men come to view infertility as a problem may become denial, when the problem persists. Looking back, Stan described how he had viewed infertility:

> When we started out, I said, 'We're older you know. We're just going to take more time [to conceive].' I would have been surprised if we got pregnant right away. So it took me quite a while before even admitting there was a problem. I considered the number of really good chances we had so low, so I would say it was a little more than a year before I realized that maybe there was a problem. And as we continued it became more clear that there really was a problem. But at the same time I still have this thing that I don't see us as really infertile and I think that there's a good chance that it can happen. I don't wipe it out completely.

Sometimes men's denial of the problem becomes extreme, as they flounder through situations with which they have never had to deal before:

> After the miscarriage, Earl said it wasn't a baby. He didn't like me calling it that. It just came a little too close. We have talked about it. We still have things to talk about. It will take some time. You can't really call it a baby, I guess.
>
> —Laurel

Men who are themselves infertile undergo a process of adjustment to loss. They sometimes become stuck in denial because there are no acceptable alternatives. Doug, who had a very low sperm count and was unwilling to try artificial insemination using a donor, said, "We just keep trying every month in the hope that one will get through."*

Occasionally, denial is taken to extremes when men cannot face their infertility. Sally and Jerry were amazed when a couple they knew underwent in vitro fertilization, even though the husband had failed the sperm penetration test.

> He wouldn't believe that no sperm penetrated. So he made his wife go through surgery, take all these hormones and drugs that you have to take. To prove a point that he never could prove.

Denial takes many different forms. It is inherent in many of the tense interactions and misunderstandings described in previous chapters. It shows up in anger, resentment, and hurt feelings directed at the partner, at the doctor, and at friends and relatives who don't understand. There may be a tendency to blame the infertility on the partner, making the partner the scapegoat for unacceptable feelings about oneself. Sitting on his couch with Sally, who was also infertile, Jerry said, "If I slept with a normal woman, I have a feeling maybe I would be fertile."

---

*The likelihood is small that conception will occur with a sperm count of less than 20 million/cc.

FACING THE LOSS

The emotional work that infertility entails is exhausting. Although enormous energy is required to maintain denial in the face of reality, equally great efforts are necessary to move on to other stages.

> I lost this sort of purposefulness, other than, 'I'm infertile.' And I have been dealing with that and not having energy for other things.
>
> —Theresa

Letting go of denial is much more than simply relinquishing the desire for a biological child. A woman must face the welter of issues surrounding her identity. Once she has begun the work of rethinking her identity, a woman becomes increasingly able to confront her infertility, and denial recedes.

> Our chances are, after all, only 50/50 that we will have children, and those aren't very good odds. And I have to live with that knowledge. I have to begin to deal with it. I have pangs I can't do this, and I feel badly that I can't, but I'm only here on earth for a short period of time. I've got a lot of other things that are satisfying.
>
> —Carrie

When women are able to face the possibility that they may not conceive, they reach a turning point. Theresa's turning point occurred after a family reunion. Surrounded by babies and pregnant relatives, her long-held subconscious fear that she would not get pregnant surfaced and suddenly seemed more real than her hopefulness. Recounting how she had driven home through the endless night in a flood of tears, she said:

> Since that weekend the odds seemed to drop a lot. I started not being able to imagine myself as pregnant. You visualize

> it, and before I could always imagine that as happening. Now I don't, I don't even imagine it. That was an awful weekend, and it took me a month to get over it. And I thought, 'Oh boy, if that was just a weekend, Christmas will be a *nightmare*.'

Women who have not succeeded in having a biological child feel as if they have been wasting their life—they have put so much energy into efforts to conceive without success. A woman who has lived this way for years feels desolate when she gives up hope, as Lisa finally did.

> I've been hooked on the technology. For years and years I've been going through this struggle but have nothing to show for it. And I'm feeling angry that I have used so much of my life and energy to deal with it. And I have nothing.
>
> Hopefully, I can make some sense out of it. I'm sure there is *some* value in it. But it's really hard to see that at this point.
>
> I feel like I might be doing some grieving. By this time in the work-up you feel pretty shattered. Infertility is so instinctual. You just follow nature's path. You just block everything else out.

When a woman begins to let go of denial and face her loss, the pain is terrible at first. She feels swamped by her feelings, which provoke a sense of inner chaos. As Laura reached the end of the work-up, she felt overwhelmed by her grief, even while she was clinging to shreds of hope:

> Nobody had ever asked me before, "What will you do if you don't get pregnant?' I immediately had visions of me failing with Pergonal the third time.* And I watched myself in my

*Pergonal, one of four brands of human menopausal gonadatropin (hMG), is a fertility drug and natural hormone made from the urine of postmenopausal women. It is an expensive drug whose use in women must be carefully supervised by a physician knowledgeable about its use. See Harkness, *The Infertility Book*, pp. 129–131.

> mind's eye falling to the ground and becoming catatonic and tears just pouring out of my face. Being completely unable to cope. I just had this instantaneous vision, and that's when I knew I was miles and miles away from accepting.
>
> And I can't get to the issue of adoption. It's on the other side of that hope. I feel like I can't get to the point of adopting until I've grieved.

Laura's inner feelings of chaos contrasted with her external sense of control over her emotions, as she struggled against the tide of grief that threatened to overwhelm her:

> I'm holding in a tremendous amount of stuff. When I was talking to you about it before, I noticed my eyes filled up a number of times. And I was surprised and thought, 'Oh, I *can* cry.' I haven't cried in seven or eight months.

Feeling Empty

Once women begin to face the loss, they feel empty. Feeling empty triggers other feelings—bitterness, negativity, desperation. Anger—sometimes rage—underlies these feelings. A woman may feel these emotions eating away at her, gnawing at her, turning life black.

Infertility affected how Angie viewed everything in life. She became concerned that she was changing as a person in negative ways, yet she felt unable to do anything to stem the tide of change:

> The thing that frightens me is, how will I resolve this? I just wonder, because I don't see my life ever being the same again.
>
> I see it affecting my life negatively. That's the only way I can see it. I'm so afraid of becoming bitter. I've never been bitter. I mean, I can be jealous, and I can be envious and competitive and all that stuff that can go into being bitter,

> that can contribute to bitterness, but it's never been an overwhelming thing for me.

Infertility affected her mood and the tenor of her daily life:

> I have been feeling really desperate. I just feel that life is worthless. I don't want to hurt myself. I wouldn't. But I don't even like feeling that black. I've done enough of torturing myself over why this is happening to me.

The inexplicable quality of infertility led to a loss of faith:

> I don't feel as blessed. I feel this disappointment with God. I want to feel that I am blessed. I mean, I am blessed, really I am. I've got so much. But it makes me feel very different from the way I used to feel.

Angie's identity was affected, even though it was Rick who was infertile. She stopped feeling special, and her world was disrupted. Reflecting on this, she said:

> I have had to face things I never had to face before. It affects your whole life, your future. I see it affecting me every day. I don't know how well I'm meeting the challenge—if I want to look at it positively as a challenge. It's a real challenge. I do see a lot of growth from it. Definitely.

She found the future hard to contemplate because she felt so overwhelmed by what infertility meant for the rest of her life:

> Whether I do or do not get pregnant, this still is going to affect my whole life. My whole outlook. The fact that I went through this. And I see that I will have to resolve this with pregnancy or something if I'm going to avoid becoming bitter.

Tangible Loss

A miscarriage, as difficult as it may be to endure, is something tangible over which to grieve. For many women, pregnancy loss initiates the grieving process, as it did for Laurel:

> For the first couple of weeks I was really up and down with my emotions, losing the baby. I thought a lot about the surgery. I thought a lot about the loss. You know, you go through the mourning. How neat it would be if it were just there, if I didn't have to go through all that.
>
> Part of me feels it was a baby. I wonder if it was a boy or girl because we really want a girl, but then another part doesn't because it is hard to visualize it as a baby because it was so small. I think, 'Where would I be now?' Then I think of when it would have been born. But I certainly thought of when it was conceived. It was either on my birthday or a couple of days after, so that is kind of neat. I don't really think of it as a dead baby, just as something that didn't quite work.

Marsha's grief, which had been locked up inside her, finally surfaced when she grieved over her dog's death. The loss of the dog translated itself into grieving for her infertility:

> Right before Christmas I started thinking about our dog who had died, and I'd say, 'My baby died,' and then I'd start to cry. You know, no matter where I was, 'My baby died, why did my baby die?' I said, 'Hal, I think I have to go to a psychiatrist because I can't stop thinking about her. I'm just not over her.' He responded, 'Well, you don't have to be Freud to realize that your baby died means your baby died.'
>
> When our terrier was still alive and we were thinking any minute we would be pregnant, I said, 'I'm so worried.

> There's no way I could love a baby as much as I love this dog,' and he said, 'Don't worry, you won't.'
>
> I find with the dog dying . . . something I loved that much—it's like a baby dying.

Some time after their dog died, Marsha and Hal got another dog. Replacing the terrier enabled Marsha to get in touch with her fears about adoption.

> Everyone said to me, 'Oh, you had to lose the other dog to get this one.' I said, 'That's fine, but I liked the other dog.'
>
> I feel the way I sense those parents at the workshop who are now adoptive parents felt when they described a child being reclaimed by the birth mother. Each one had a previous adopted child who had been reclaimed—one at three months, one at one week, one at the hospital. Two have since adopted. All of them said, 'Well, of course it was worthwhile because now we have this wonderful baby.' But it didn't make it all worthwhile, the way they talked about it. They cried.

Women may fear that once they begin to express their grief, it will be endless. They sense the depths of their grief, and it seems bottomless. They fear it will be their undoing. As supportive as Hal was about Marsha's need to grieve, she was apprehensive about the cycle of grief starting again, and how it would affect her emotionally, as well as its potential effect on their relationship:

> I know it's going to start over again, the same way I felt in December when I was crying all the time. I started again today. It's the anniversary of the terrier's death. And my brother phoned to say he and his new wife are pregnant.

Theresa felt immobilized by her grief for a long period of time, which led to depression and inertia:

> I'm doing okay right now. My experience has been that around the corner you can get real blue and melancholy. And when I do, I think, 'Oh my God . . .' you know, losing it again.

It's important to feel fully all the emotions running through you. This helps to cleanse the wound. But by the same token, it's important not to let your feelings take over for so long that they get the better of you. When mourning goes on and on, women and men become immobilized by it.

Infertility has had its turn running your life. Sooner or later it's time to wrest yourself out of its clutches and go on with your life.

MEN'S EXPERIENCE OF LOSS

Men experience loss just as women do but because of cultural rules about men not being emotionally expressive, their response to infertility may seem much more muted.

> In Resolve the men don't do nearly as much talking. And a lot of them, I know for a fact, have their own problem, but they don't talk much, either. It's a real, real difficult thing for a man.
>
> —Angie

Biological differences between men and women and the expectations they hold account for some of the difference in response.

> There was a reassessing of what was going on, and we got involved in a fertility program. And also I was worried about Sandra's age. She was getting toward the end of child-bearing. I think that it was hard to come to terms with that, to accept that she was at the end of her potential child-bearing time. To give it up, to accept that, was harder on her

> than on me. Though I have some hard feelings about it. A sense of loss.
>
> —Tony

Sometimes men feel there is no place for them in the grieving process. They feel left out.

> I guess I want to share in the grieving a little bit. I don't want it to be all on Susan. Seeing her in pain like that hurts me. And some of those feelings are irrespective of infertility.
>
> —Larry

Men who are infertile may demonstrate a more acute sense of loss than men who are not because they must mourn the loss of their reproductive ability. Sometimes they become immobilized by their sense of loss:

> I can see how people get so overwhelmed by depression. It's real hard to get up in the morning. I mean, I hate it. I used to love it. I used to go running, I used to do so many things.
>
> —Jerry

When Matt and Jenny attempted to adopt and the birth mother changed her mind, Matt experienced conflicting feelings as he acknowledged the loss the child stood for:

> I was euphoric when she changed her mind. I was relieved that this potential symbol of my inability to be a father was gone. I still think about it. I still feel the pain, and that's something I will probably always feel.

Matt associated his sense of loss with failure.

> I don't take failure well. I never have, I never will. And that was one of my major failures in life that I will have to live with. Even today, I'll be walking down the street and see some little kid and I flash back.

CHILDREN AND LOSS

If a couple has children, facing the loss means their children will face it, too. Their feelings about the loss may affect the child. Penny and George, who had one child after several years of infertility and were trying to have another, were unprepared for the effect infertility had on their daughter. Penny said:

> When we talk about our infertility, we can't ignore the effect on our daughter. When she was 5, she went through a really bad time, and it's hard for me to get a grip on whether I was overreacting and encouraging her behavior or not. But she seemed to be very depressed. She talked a lot about going in the middle of the street and wanting to get run over. Things like that. That disturbed me a lot from things I had read that a 5-year-old doesn't understand the permanence of death.
>
> We consulted a child psychologist. The basic message was that we had involved her too much in our feelings, you know, the roller coaster of emotions, and that she was getting the message that she wasn't enough. She wasn't adequate, and that was too much of a burden for her to handle.

George interjected:

> Which was probably true. Of course, it's not anything you do intentionally. It's just everyday. You don't hide your moods from your kid. They probably know them better than anybody else.

Penny continued:

> And I'd had surgery, and all the things that were physically debilitating. So I think she was worried about my health as

> well, and she was very needy. There's no doubt about that. The crisis more or less helped me to get a better grasp on how to deal with the infertility. At least not letting it hang out all the time and being more conscientious and consistent with her as far as my moods were concerned.
>
> And also giving her the power to confront me with my own emotions. About that time on our refrigerator we had a sign that changed: 'Mom's mood is good,' and 'Mom's mood is bad,' and it was hers. She was the one who manipulated it. It was kind of her signal to us. She doesn't use it much anymore, but for a while it was constantly changing.

THE EFFECTS OF OTHER LIFE CRISES

The death of a loved one in the midst of infertility not only makes infertility tangible, it magnifies the loss. The future becomes difficult to contemplate because it now seems finite: people are dying, yet children are not being born to replace them in the flow of generations. At least this is the way it seems. Laurel's miscarriage brought up old grief about her mother's death, which had occurred just before she began trying to conceive:

> After my mom died I went to a support group and it helped, but nobody's ever going to bring her back. So it's just something you have to deal with. I was trying to work through that.

Women and men sometimes link their emotional response to infertility to deaths among the older generation. They may be especially affected by the death of childless relatives. Dying without having children is often viewed as an interruption to the ongoing cycle of life, a discontinuity they fear will be echoed in their own lives.

> I got the check today from my aunt's estate. There's something that is really disturbing about being 62 years old without children. You know, she left nothing behind her.
>
> —Sally

Someone's death may precipitate grief and depression. When men experience the death of a loved one, they may find themselves in a crisis:

> For a couple of years it was real stressful because his dad developed cancer, and he was dying—this was in the Midwest. We would take little mini-vacations here, but we had to use most of our vacation time to go back and deal with that. It was horrible that we had to go there because we had to see everybody. It was pretty sad and distressful. That issue was a difficult thing to deal with during the infertility, too. That, combined with the infertility, has really taken a toll on him. I know it has. He went into therapy after his dad died.
>
> —Lisa

Infertility often occurs as people are approaching mid-life. Mid-life has been characterized as a time when individuals first face their own eventual mortality, as their parents grow old. During the time they are dealing with feelings of emptiness over their infertility, women and men often express a preoccupation with death and the finiteness of life that is part of the work of coming to terms with their own eventual mortality.

The deaths of others prompts reflection on the meaning of life.

> When someone dies, you begin to live with it, and then you learn from it, and then you grow. And then you go on, and it is done. And you have to live with it. Infertility isn't like that.
>
> —Angie

> I started to realize that I'm pretty young, and this is just the beginning. I don't like thinking about that but what are you going to do? You can't just isolate yourself and not have any relationships and be bitter. We don't really have a choice. We're here on earth, and we do the best we can.
>
> —Laurel

When men and women are able to get in touch with their feelings, they take *the* major step toward healing. Infertility is a catalyst in reckoning with the issues of mid-life, as women and men not only put their fertility into perspective, they examine the meaning of their entire life. In the search for answers, they may find greater unity in their relationship. And in themselves.

CHAPTER 9

SEEKING UNITY

When a couple reaches the point where they can identify infertility as a mutual enemy, rather than as a fault lurking in one of them, they become united in their efforts.

> Ned said to me, 'You know, I'm not going to Resolve because I need to go. I'm doing it because I think it will help me about 25 percent, and I want to be there for you and help you with driving and talk with you.'
>
> So it feels really good. That's one thing about our relationship that is really good. After all the adversity and hard part, it does bring you closer together, because it's you and me against the infertile bug. So we've got that kind of bonding. That's really nice. I feel really secure about that.
>
> —Donna

It is nice. Once a couple has this, they have an unshakeable bond, forged in steel, that will see them through anything. A bond that will add depth and breadth to their relationship. The question is, How does a couple get to this place?

This kind of unity doesn't happen overnight. It is a slow process that occurs over time, as both partners take stock of the situation and its effect on their relationship. And because partners seldom identify a problem at the same time and proceed in synchrony with each other, getting to the point of feeling united against the foe—the fertility problem—usually does take time. Sometimes it takes a long time.

We can best understand how to move toward unity by looking at the different kinds of dynamics that affect the relationship.

These are of two sorts. The first set of dynamics is each individual's intrapsychic processes—everything that goes on inside a person, whether it is consciously experienced or not. This includes all of those identity issues that revolve around masculinity and femininity.

The second set of dynamics are those that take place between partners—not just their interactions with each other and their actions as a team, but everything they bring to the relationship—their thoughts, feelings, and their past experiences from the family in which they were raised. When two people come together, they each bring their self and all its accoutrements to the relationship. In doing so, they perpetuate their family system.

There is an ongoing debate among practitioners and social scientists about whether relationship issues should be approached via individual dynamics or by examining a couple's life together as a family system. In this book we explore both levels because each one is essential to see the whole picture clearly. Looking at one level without looking at the other is like looking out of a pair of glasses that has only one lens—half the visual field will be murky. This is why, to reach a unified approach to the relationship, we need to look at ourselves as individuals as well. In order to effectively seek unity with each other, it is also necessary to seek unity in oneself.

DIFFERENTIATING ONESELF FROM THE PARTNER

Knowing who we are as a person helps us to understand how we live out our part in the relationship. By gaining more clarity about ourself—our wants, needs, feelings—we will be better able to communicate them to our partner. The more insight we have into our inner self, the better able we will be to see ourself as a separate person and determine our needs as an individual.

And this is important. When we can see ourself as a separate being, the less likely we will be to assign the parts of us that we have a hard time living with to our partner to live out for us. These are the parts of ourselves we are uncomfortable with, feel bad about, or don't like. Assigning the disavowed parts of ourself—the angry, or impetuous, or rigid parts—to our partner is a process called projective identification. It is a part of every relationship, no matter how healthy. At best, we can work hard at not handing over our emotional baggage to each other. At worst, we can drown each other with it, and ultimately fail to have any idea whatsoever of who the other person really is. For most of us, the way we see our partner lies somewhere in the middle of these two poles.

What is a projection? Very simply, a projection is a misjudgment we make about another person. But unlike a common error of judgment, a projection is hard to correct because we are emotionally invested in the perception behind the projection. For example, how many times have we met someone for the first time who is familiar in some positive way? We may jump to conclusions about what that individual is like as a person. If, much later, we find out just how different that person really is from whom we imagined him or her to be, we may become depressed, disillusioned, and even angry at that individual for not living up to our expectations. This is a projection.

Once a projection is riddled with holes, it may be discarded, or it may come to life again every time we interact with, or think about, that person. It depends on the power of the original association as well as on the importance of that individual in our life.

The same phenomenon is at work when it comes to choosing a partner. We don't choose just anybody. We choose a person who is familiar—perhaps very familiar—in the same way, but we can't put our finger on what is so familiar. Usually we choose someone we are comfortable with—someone we feel at home with—someone who seems to know us well, who makes a good fit with us. Even if our partner seems exotically different at first, there is usually something—something indefinable—that we are comfortable with.

How is it that we choose someone who is such a good fit, who seems to really know us? Partly, it's because our partner chose us for an identical set of reasons, and, as a result, we are familiar to each other. We are well known, to some extent. Our partner may be like a family member from our original family. Or perhaps our partner isn't like any one person but instead carries an amalgam of traits from that first, so important, family group. Even if what we wanted in choosing a mate was to put distance between ourselves and that original family, we somehow aren't able to do it. The lure of the known, and yet unknown, is too great.

It's the unknown part of this equation that ultimately causes some difficulty. Because we fill in our own ideas about the unknown part of our partner. And our ideas are based on our past experience.

These are the roots of projection.

One of the most difficult things for Laura to deal with during her infertility treatment was her feeling that she had no acceptable outlet for her emotions. She likened Stan's discomfort about her emotionality to her family's distaste for her behavior when she was a child.

> Stan is uncomfortable when I'm emotional. This whole thing has been a replay of my experience as a kid. I'm sure this is related to the dynamic of my home when I was a child. 'Laura causes all the problems. Laura gets hysterical. If only Laura didn't get angry at her mother, or burst into tears over something, we'd have a perfectly happy home. What is it with Laura?' And there's a bit of that in this relationship, too. Although Stan is much more tolerant, much less into browbeating me. But he is uncomfortable with it.

Laura is a step ahead of many people because she can, at least, see similarities between her relationship with Stan and her other family relationships, especially with her mother. But what she—and most of us—can't see when we are engulfed by any issue that is linked to our identity is how our own and our partner's responses trigger a replay of the original scenario. All of the feelings—the anger, the sense of rejection, the loneliness, the frustration, the despair—everything that was present in those early encounters wells up again in the current relationship. Each interaction, every interchange, may become charged with emotions from the past that have simply lain dormant until now.

And now Stan and Laura are in their forties and trying to deal with their fertility issues. Stan, less self-involved in the problem, makes a simple response to something Laura says, and if it isn't exactly the right tone, or doesn't reflect her own sentiments, it undergoes a metamorphosis into those charged scenes from her childhood home. Soon he has become the bad guy, the unfeeling, aloof husband—at least in her eyes.

This is exactly what happened in their relationship.

This is why it is important to try to withdraw our projections from each other. Because so many of the misunderstandings and hurt feelings that partners experience in the relationship revolve around misjudgments about who the other person is, and about questions that arise concerning the nature of their intentions.

Learning to identify our projections and then to withdraw them is, at best, an arduous task. Of all the difficult endeavors we face in life, it is one of the hardest. And one that never ends. But when fertility is the issue, it is an important goal to work toward—and work it is—as is any issue in an intimate relationship. Projections are aided and abetted by the expectations that revolve around gender. And gender, we have painfully come to realize, is loaded enough on its own.

To begin to sort out the issues in your relationship, you need to first untangle yourself from your partner. Start by trying to step outside yourself and look at yourself and your partner as two individuals. This may not be so easy to do, especially if you have been together a long time, or see yourselves as knitted together in a symbiotic way. Keep your own gender clearly in mind as you explore your inner self. Think about how your own and your partner's experience is shaped differently by your gender. You will find that many of the hurts you may carry from interactions between you that went amiss dissolve when you consider yourselves in the broader context in which you live—the culture.

Culture is a lofty and abstract term. If trying to envision the effects of culture on you and your partner as female and male stops you in your tracks, break this idea down into small, digestible pieces. Try thinking about how you and your partner are affected by stereotypes of the real man and woman, or differences in how you and your partner were socialized, or how your roles are different.

Then try to compare and contrast yourself with your partner in a nonjudgmental way. Have you lost your empathy for your partner in this struggle? If you have, try thinking about what the world may be like through his or her eyes. What issues come up when you put fertility on the table for discussion? Who brings up what? What doesn't get talked about? Does either of you have nagging concerns? Other problems that won't go away?

The more clearly you are able to see yourself and your partner, the more clearly you will see that behavior that appears to be directed at you—behavior over which you may have hurt feelings—is really triggered by the situation and isn't meant for you at all. Your partner may be dealing with issues that revolve around his own gender identity. Or he may be responding to issues of the self. Perhaps he has hurt feelings from some previous encounter and is reacting to you rather than acting on his own behalf. In other words, carryover from some previous exchanges between you may be occurring, or from another relationship, as Laura's and Stan's family ghosts were often included in their interchanges.

Issues surrounding the self crop up continually in intimate relationships, so the trigger that sets off difficulties between you may be a replay of something that happened long ago, before you met. When you work at this together, you can diminish the number of projections that may fly back and forth between you, and see each other for who you really are.

OVERCOMING THREATS TO THE SELF

It is rare for two individuals to change at precisely the same rate and in the same way. Consequently, the sense of synchrony between partners that lends an aura of stability to their relationship may be temporarily lost during the time one or both of them is experiencing change. Much as a 6-year-old undergoes a growth spurt upon entering a new world in the first grade, so does a 36-year-old who is facing an onslaught of mid-life issues, especially if the prospect is great that this life stage may differ from what was anticipated.

Any unexpected event in life presents us with opportunity, even an event we view as a tragedy. It pushes our limits, it shoves us out of our comfortable little world—to grow, to change—to become more fully ourselves and make the most of our potential in life. But it also poses a threat—to the known, expectable world in which we live.

The situation you and your partner find yourselves in creates the threat. And the threat is to the self—the most central part of our personhood. We experience this threat through our gender identity. Each of us feels this threat—as a man, as a woman.

The issues become confused in living with this dilemma on an everyday basis. They get mixed up with other concerns in the relationship. And then the threat to the self grows. And we react to the threat out of fear, rather than acting on behalf of who we are and what we need as an individual.

Susan, talking with Larry, described how she felt when she was out of synchrony with him:

> It became a source of strain between us. Here I was feeling and experiencing something and felt like you didn't even think it existed. So it was like a complete contradiction of reality. You look for other people to validate your reality.
>
> It means that I'm crazy in a way, like, 'Here's something that I see so clearly that the person most close to me in my life and closely involved in it doesn't see at all. I must be crazy.'

Susan was experiencing something called cognitive dissonance—when two pieces of reality don't fit together. When the issue is fertility, different realities often become opposing camps represented by oneself and one's partner. Susan, trying to resist the threat she felt from the idea that she might be crazy, was clinging to her inner core of knowledge about herself, that she was not crazy. And since she knew she was not, she had been able to hold her own so far without getting lost in the threat to her self. She believed she had been forthrightly expressing her feelings about their fertility issues for over a year, but felt she had been getting almost no response from Larry.

Why not? How did Larry view the problem? This is how he responded to what Susan said:

> When we were working overseas we decided we were going to try again when we came home. We sort of renewed our pledge to each other to try and work together the next time we went through the work-up, so that we wouldn't be at cross-purposes. So since we've come back, I have been trying to get more involved myself.
>
> I guess I felt not as much a part of the process before. Susan always answered my questions. But because you're so close to the situation, it's like you won't let yourself believe it or you don't know how to try to sort it out. Sometimes you need somebody you don't know telling you things before you believe them.
>
> We weren't getting any of that. There was just no contact with the doctor at all. It was like it was all Susan's problem.
>
> We didn't talk about infertility that much and so it took a while to come to the point where we were focused on it together.

Larry's response—an orderly, historical approach to their current situation—is a far cry from Susan's view of two realities that don't jibe, that make her feel crazy. What is happening here? Larry has distanced himself from the problem out of fear—a reaction to the threat to the self. He has taken on the attitude that their fertility problem didn't have much to do with him. This attitude was reinforced in the health care setting that Susan was being treated in, where physicians did not see women together with their partners, or include men in any other way.*

What needs to change? How can Susan and Larry, now that they are talking about it, get on the same wavelength? In order to create unity in this situation, the answer is fairly straightforward but not necessarily easy to accomplish. Larry needs to let go of his distance, his disavowal of any part in this problem, and instead embrace the problem equally with Susan.

What is happening inside this man that prevents him from doing this?

He is feeling threatened. Life as he knows it is in jeopardy. Something has gone awry with the relationship, and he has retreated. He is emotionally unavailable. But he is not tuned out. He is immobilized with fear. And proceeding with caution.

Even though Larry doesn't have an infertility factor himself, his experience of infertility is just as primal as that faced by men who do have a fertility problem. Because it is an indirect threat to another male role—the expectation that a man can establish and keep a successful marital relationship. When the ability to do so appears to be in jeopardy, it affects a man's gender identity, just as the gender identity of a man who is infertile is affected by the threat to his masculinity. When a man is able to acknowledge the threat to the relationship, his self-involvement in the problem begins to equal that of his partner.

We all have our own characteristic responses to threat. Some people respond passively to threats by retreating, while others attack. Although an attack may appear to be motivated by anger, the underlying emotion is fear. Still others become immobilized and unable to move in any direction—they become literally frozen with fear.

A threat may be vague and amorphous, or it may be concrete.

---

*Although it is commonly stated in treatment for infertility that "the couple is the patient," this philosophy is not realized in many health care settings. It is therefore important for couples to assertively follow this rule of thumb in seeking health care. The initial physician or clinic visit is of particular importance. Both partners should attend it and any subsequent talks or decision-making meetings with the practitioner.

Sometimes the threat becomes menacing. It seems to be everywhere. Then it recedes, and we can't grasp what it was about. We can't put our finger on exactly what was so threatening. Life goes back to normal. Until the threat materializes again. Eventually, we begin to have insight about what we find threatening, and why we react as we do. But insight doesn't usually come in full force until we disarm the threat—until we dust the cobwebs off it and look it full in the face—until we dismantle it and see it for what it is. As only a threat, not reality.

A man needs to uncover his feelings, to jump in and get involved. Life as he knows it is at stake. Until he can recognize an inner voice saying, "This is scary," and acknowledge what it means, he will continue to distance himself. And he will continue to feel the threat to the relationship.

Tony pondered why he had become withdrawn in response to Sandra's increased demands. In part, he felt overwhelmed by her purposefulness. When a man observes his partner's single-minded purpose in full swing, he may feel in danger of being blotted out by it. This is the threat of engulfment.

> At times I have felt that she wanted children and a family so much that I was almost secondary, that I was a means to get that. She was getting older, and feeling a little desperate, and I felt she was pushing our relationship along in that respect, and that made me withdraw somewhat.

This combination of threats—abandonment and engulfment—is just as great as the threat infertility poses for a man's masculinity. Even though they are usually felt as muted or remote, these, too, are threats to the self. Because abandonment and engulfment are two poles of the same continuum, the person feeling threatened is torn between two opposing sets of feelings—"Don't leave me!" and "Don't get too close!"

> And there is my own emotional stuff in growing up and facing being an adult, and that kind of thing. I thought I dealt with it when we started the relationship, but there is more.
>
> —Tony

SORTING OUT GRIEF FROM ANGER

Sometimes couples successfully manage infertility for years at a time, only to have the relationship become vulnerable and nearly succumb to the grief and anger infertility provokes. With hindsight, Abby told the story of how she had unconsciously tried to sabotage her relationship with John, a relationship that was formerly very close and caring:

> We went on a very short vacation up to the lake and had a really nice time. We really needed that break. I didn't want to come back because I didn't want to deal with the infertility. But we did come back, and it was really a letdown after this wonderful time that we had had. I began to grieve over our infertility like I had never grieved before. It was like no other grief I had experienced up to that point. It was like an all-consuming, total grief. I was really grieving the child we couldn't have. So here I was emoting.
>
> I became furious at John for not grieving in the same way, for him being so contained and calm. What happened was, it started driving us apart. I couldn't be angry at him for being infertile. His infertility was not his fault. But I could be angry at him for everything else he did to hurt me, so I went on this rampage! I went back to the beginning of our relationship: 'If you hadn't done this, this wouldn't have happened. How dare you!' It was a rampage. That's how I was dealing with my grief. That started to drive a wedge between us.
>
> So when I was ready to move on with the next phase of infertility treatment, John said, 'I'm not ready,' and that was the last straw for me. Then it became, 'You stand in the way of everything. You're depriving me.' I had no control, no power. So I threatened divorce, almost.

John interjected, "She saw me as withholding from her. And as holding all the cards."

Abby resumed,

> I heard him say, 'I can't do this,' instead of 'I can't do it this month, and I might not be able to do it next month.' I interpreted it as 'I'm not going to give this to you,' and so my feeling was, 'Well, if this is what you're going to do, then I don't know if I can stay married to you. Because if you don't give me this, I don't know how I'll ever be able to stay with you.' I didn't hear him say, 'It's just not for right now.' I was desperate to have a kid at that point.
>
> So it was really, really bad there for a while. I had no empathy for him. I couldn't understand him, and I was misinterpreting him, and as soon as I would start in, he would get defensive, of course, so he couldn't allay any of my fears. I was desperate. Finally, we had a truce. We took a vacation and we didn't talk about it at all. And every time we started talking about it, we had a fight. We just couldn't talk about it . . . *at all*! During those eight weeks I was trying to convince myself that life would be okay if we didn't have children because I was just assuming that we wouldn't have any. In defense, I was trying to convince myself that I'd find other things to do, and 'Who wants this, anyway?'
>
> Then after that, it took us a while to get back on track and start talking again. I realized how unreasonable I had been. So when we came back and we had a few discussions, and then he decided not too long ago to go forward, and, well, he's ambivalent, I'm ambivalent, but that's the way it is, and you're not going to be 100 percent sure, and nobody we talked to was. You just know you don't want to be without children. So that's where we are now. Although we decided, I feel a sense of inertia. I just can't get up the motivation to actually proceed.

Abby and John survived Abby's assault on the relationship because they had developed a strong relationship over the years they had been together and because they had always worked together on their infertility. Most of all, however, their relationship survived this assault because Abby came to her senses and recognized her destructive behavior before it was too late. Once they were able to start talking to each other again, they were gradually able to surmount this impasse and move on.

They went on to talk about other things, and later on in the interview I came back to it:

> Gay: It sounds like you've sort of gotten past that time where you were fighting a lot. You talk about it like it's in the past. Is that so?
>
> Abby: Well, I feel like that episode is in the past. Yeah, I feel like that was a chapter. I think we're still recovering, though. I still think it's a very difficult thing for us to talk about.
>
> John: I think we're scarred and so beat up from this whole process. It has happened to so many couples. We're scarred.
>
> Abby: Yeah, plus with John's unemployment and job search, and all of that on top of everything. He's got this job now, but they don't have an office for him. He's up in the air with that. When we got married we didn't know we were going to go through this, and it's sort of a feeling of disillusionment. This isn't what I bargained for. I had a dream, and this wasn't it. So I think there is a lot of that going on, too.

CHAPTER 10

WORKING TOGETHER

A complex emotional process is triggered when family members make the transition from one phase of life to the next. As their relationship develops, partners establish patterns that form the basis for the ongoing development of the family system in their generation. But when partners prepare to move into the next stage of life, they experience growth and change as individuals that, in turn, affects the patterns they have developed in their family system.

A family system may run efficiently, regardless of how healthy it is, as long as the status quo is maintained. Even a faulty system may run smoothly if it is not disturbed. But when an event occurs that threatens the system with change, the system loses its efficiency. A period of upheaval follows, in which questions and issues are raised that directly or indirectly threaten its existence. Many events can, and do, threaten a family system, by provoking changes in individual roles and identity. This is what happens when a fertility problem occurs.

Infertility is an event that threatens the future of the family. It questions the very existence of the family system by potentially interrupting the flow of generations. The discovery of a fertility problem triggers two kinds of stress in the family system—stress that may potentially affect the functioning of any family, no matter what the issues are. The first kind of stressors are those that come down to us over the generations, and include family myths and expectations, such as attitudes about having children. The second sort are stressors that affect the family as it moves through time, dealing with life-cycle transitions and unexpected events in life. Family clinicians Elizabeth Carter and Monica

McGoldrick have observed that when the two types of stress intersect, there is a surge in the amount of anxiety generated in the family. The greater the anxiety created at any transition point, the more difficult that transition will be.

THE ROOTS OF STRESS

When the family life cycle is suddenly thrown off course, strain appears in the relationship. At first it is insidious, unexpectedly cropping up here and there. If the source of strain persists, it may become pervasive, burrowing into the vulnerable parts of the relationship and taking root.

When partners experience growth and change as individuals that is not reflected in their family system, they experience growing pains in their relationship. When one partner changes and the other one lags behind, or when partners change in different ways, these growing pains may become intense as they attempt to refocus the family system to mesh more effectively with their individual changes. This is not an easy task. There is no ready antidote for these incongruities. The best medicine is to work together on retuning the partnership to reflect each person's new level of personal development. Otherwise, one partner may be left behind. And both partners may become alienated from each other.

Casting about to find a culprit on which to pin the responsibility for added stress in the partnership, women and men may focus on their differences to the exclusion of other issues. Fertility issues go straight to the center of a woman's or man's identity. It is not necessary for partners to actually live out stereotypic roles in their life together to feel that somehow being male, or being female, has suddenly become an underlying issue in the relationship. Different approaches to the problem cause an imbalance between partners that emotionally loads the way they relate to each other. For example, when one partner seeks to solve the problem through action while the other partner wants to avoid it, stress and conflict ensue.

> I was always the pusher. I guess the real change happened when I stopped being the only pusher, and we started working more together. That's when the problem became bearable—when we were a couple working on it as opposed to two separate people. That's when it was bearable. When we weren't, it was unbearable.
>
> —Celia

Gender differences camouflage deeper issues if partners stereotype each other. For example, if a woman explains her husband's silence about infertility to herself as being a typically uninvolved man, and a man discounts his partner's concerns by telling himself she is a hysterical woman, a barrier is created. Stereotypes lead partners away from each other—away from talking about their fears and intangible anxieties. Rationales such as, "There's no point in talking about it—he/she wouldn't understand, anyway," are self-defeating and obscure the real issues.

While polarization may appear to occur along gender lines, an underlying set of cultural attributes present in the relationship contributes much more significantly to the development of stress between partners. These attributes include power, innocence, competence, responsibility, trust, and the expression of feelings. These are some of the major ones—there are undoubtedly more. They reflect core American values—the ideals we espouse in our daily lives. These values include achievement and success, activity and work, individualism, competence and control, progress, and an orientation toward the future.

The family is a mainstay for the perpetuation of culture. Families internalize these cultural values and incorporate them into family themes and in individual family members' identity issues. Gender may be an issue within each of them. For example, when a woman's ability to manage the family checkbook is questioned, gender is implicit in issues of power and competence.

The emphasis placed on cultural values in family interactions gives them their emotional charge, an emphasis that is lived out over and over again in the family.

> You come to a point in your life where you have to ask yourself, 'Do I believe this because I believe it or because I was raised to believe it?' You have to decide your own morals, values, priorities in life. How are you going to spend your time? How are you going to spend your money? How are you going to raise kids? We dealt with that. 'Well, we did it this way in my family's home. Do we have to do it that way again?' You have to decide.
>
> —Sheila

The likelihood is great that those qualities that most affect the dynamics of a couple's relationship percolated in each partner's original family group, as well. So accustomed are we to the familiar and well known that we are often blind about behavior that has always been part of our world. For example, if issues of power and competence clouded communication in the family we started life in, the likelihood is great that we will bring those issues with us into our partnership, no matter how differently they may manifest themselves now. The phenomenon of hand-me-down dynamics gives them a density that renders them hard to fathom.

Driven by the need to successfully make the next transition in the family life cycle, women and men stumble over the invisible, yet ever-present, values embedded in their relationship. In the relationship, these values become expressions of personal identity for each partner, an identity that—in the heat of a problem—feels challenged. Take, for example, two of the most frequently fought-about topics among American couples: money and sex. What are the underlying issues? Most often, they have to do with the same dimensions, especially power, competence, responsibility, and trust—issues that directly reflect American values—

being competent, taking responsibility, learning to trust and be trustworthy.

Linking these values back to personal identity issues, and to cultural expectations men and women attempt to live out, it is easy to see why seemingly simple issues have the potential to launch the relationship into a sea of seething emotions by threatening both individuals and their partnership at every level. The clarity and objectivity partners must struggle toward may, for a time, be completely lost from view.

In the scheme of daily life, each attribute of the relationship that reflects cultural values has a continuum, along which both partners move, shifting from one place to another, as they go through life together. If the relationship becomes polarized, partners may find themselves at opposite poles on every dimension that manifests itself in their relationship. Polarization in the relationship can slow down—and even destroy—a couple's ability to become united.

POLARIZATION

What leads to polarization? Ideally, partners will succeed in balancing each of the dimensions in their relationship between them. But balance is hard to achieve. In the process of projective identification, unconscious agreement may have occurred between a man and a woman about any or all of their relational qualities. The way that partners divide these qualities between them depends on what each individual brings to the relationship and the unconscious agreements they make about who is responsible for the expression of specific emotions and roles within the family.

She, for example, may have taken on the expression of anger for both partners because showing anger is a near impossibility for him. Anger may seldom have been directly expressed in his family, even though anger may have been a funnel for other emotions, such as fear, in hers. The same couple may also have worked out who will express responsibility when problems arise. If it's hard for her to acknowledge any responsibility for their problems, he may take on the role of placater and express feelings of guilt and failure for her as well as for himself.

Once a pattern of interaction is established, it may polarize the relationship. As time passes, her expressions of anger may multiply and be directed increasingly at him. Even though he is expressing feelings of failure for both of them, she is conscious only of her growing frustration with his seeming incompetence. He, in turn, feels increasingly like a failure because she is so angry. He thinks, "There must be a reason—it must be justified." Her anger reinforces his feelings of worthlessness, while his expression of failure reinforces her need to be perfect—to cover up the cracks in the relationship that might be her responsibility.

In time, everything else feeds into these two caricatures they have created of each other. Can someone who wants to believe she is perfect live with someone who thinks he is worthless? They can, and they do, but not happily.

The pattern partners develop together may be a replication of patterns in their original families. In this particular instance, angry self-righteousness pits itself against apologetic self-effacement. These stances within the relationship may reflect roles that partners observed their parents enacting when they themselves were children. Why does role repetition occur so frequently across generations? Because the family system encompasses several generations. Parents and other important relatives are role models. As dysfunctional and unrewarding as some roles learned in the family may be, they are often the only ones we know.

Drifting Toward Opposite Poles

Not every relationship becomes polarized. But when an unexpected event, such as infertility, occurs, the bombardment partners feel from multiple stresses may create "drift" toward different poles until they are able to sort out and untangle the different elements affecting the relationship.

One way that drift occurs is through unconscious conspiracy between partners. A man may want to avoid having to deal with infertility, while his partner may have low expectations for the role he should take. Like many couples, Theresa and Paul drifted into unintentional collusion, with Theresa soft-pedaling her concerns and feelings.

> Sometimes you cash in and say, 'It's important to me. I'd really like you to go if you can.' But you worry about being too pushy.

Why is this cashing in? Why is this being pushy? This is a reasonable expectation—that both partners will participate in family concerns. Fertility issues involve both partners.

When a woman excuses her partner from taking part in the relationship, she helps to perpetuate the situation. She feels abandoned, and if she decides she must handle the problem alone, she becomes a martyr. If she allows her partner to stay in retreat, his retreat may eventually become a sort of semipermanent retirement from the life of the family. Not only will it affect the outcome of this issue, a pattern may jell for everything that follows in their future life together, as well.

Polarization around gender is the dominant pattern in partnerships when fertility is an issue. This is not the only pattern of polarization that may develop. There are others, and the potential for a deadlock to occur with other patterns is just as great. But polarization along gender lines is by far the most common one partners are ensnared by.

They become caught in this net because the problem poses a threat to their gender identity. Gender may therefore be the "hook" on which the relationship gets snagged. But it is not the heart of the issue.

Laurel and Earl have a family system that appears to revolve around gender issues. To all appearances she is the needy female and he is the stoic, remote male. The reality is much different, however.

> Earl came and picked me up after the laparoscopy, so he got to meet the doctor and talk with him. But it has pretty much been my campaign. I joined a Resolve support group and I went to that alone.* He doesn't feel the need to talk about it. It's not affecting him. One time I asked him if he would give me the shots [for hMG]. And he said, 'No way!' He is a little bit squeamish. I paint him as a bad guy but he is not really.
>
> Sometimes I am sorry he doesn't go to the Resolve group. You kind of feel left out when you are the only single one. Earl would never go. Well, maybe I never asked him. Maybe I just assumed that he wouldn't want to go.

What is happening here? Not only is Laurel living out the role of caretaker and allowing Earl to take the role of spoiled child, she is protecting him from having to confront himself or deal with the problems of life. She is giving him a message, "It's okay if you don't grow up." Acting childlike is a very ineffective way of dealing with infertility. It is only when we become grounded in our self as an adult that we can recognize and acknowledge that, as vulnerable as we feel, we need to be responsible adults in dealing with infertility.

When partners unconsciously conspire with each other so that one partner is absolved of taking a responsible adult role, that person becomes a perennial child. Earl is stuck. He can't grow up and acknowledge acting childlike—his fears and his vulnerability—until he and Laurel unlock their conspiracy that has polarized the relationship.

Without any kind of incentive to look inside himself, or get in touch with what is happening in their life together, Earl simply

*Every Resolve chapter sponsors support groups. Although partners are encouraged to attend as a couple, women also attend these meetings without their partner.

withdraws further. From his point of view, it's safer if there is no change in their relationship. If Laurel has no expectations, he's not going to volunteer any changes. Because change might upset the status quo.

In their case, it's up to Laurel to stop making excuses for him—to cease to make life so comfortable, enabling him to just coast along. Most people, given the opportunity to skip the hard parts in life, will take it. Earl is no exception. Laurel, meanwhile, struggling alone in the martyr role, is not being honest with herself or with Earl. She is shortchanging both of them.

What would happen if she sat down one day, looked him square in the eye, and said, "Look, this is a crisis. I had a miscarriage—our baby died. I am still mourning my mother's death. I am fighting with the insurance company every day, and trying to do my job, even though I can't concentrate. And here you sit, watching TV day and night, and only allowing me to bring up these issues when the TV is on. This has to stop. Are you in this relationship, or aren't you? I need your help. I need your support. I can't do it any longer on my own. I'm not going to make excuses for you anymore. I have had it. Wake up."

What do you think would happen?

If you are a woman who is protecting her man from knowing himself—from growing up and having to deal with life—think again. Why are you doing this? Is it because you need to keep the control in the relationship, albeit quietly and unobtrusively? Or is it because you are trying to protect the relationship? Either way, it isn't going to work. You may make it through infertility without rocking the boat—maybe—but you can't make it through your whole life together doing it this way. It's this dynamic that eventually makes women wild with anger and men feel like innocent victims.

The Fear Factor

Possibly one of the most astute comments ever made by a politician was Franklin Delano Roosevelt's, "The only thing we have to fear is fear itself." Fear is a potent element in intimate relationships. One of its most lethal aspects is its ability to boomerang, to contaminate intimacy and turn on the self.

Women and men try not to rock the boat in an intimate relationship because of the fear factor. We fear that the tiniest added stress will unravel the relationship. We hang back, opting for comfort in the short-term as opposed to satisfaction and togetherness in the long-term.

But it's a false comfort and an exaggerated fear. If the relationship as it stands has a glimmer of unreality because one or both partners' needs are not being met, that's cold comfort. And if either partner expects that a single pressure point will be the relationship's undoing, the strength of the partnership is being underestimated. If a relationship is really so weak that one partner must pump all the air into the other to keep it afloat, it may not be possible to salvage anyway. Most often, fears about the relationship's weak links are not real. They are simply fears, and nothing more.

Fears feed polarization. They prevent partners from speaking up, from saying whatever is pressing up from within—communiqués from the self that need to come forth, to hang in the air, if necessary.

Fear prevents communication. Left alone, fear grows. It leads to something worse—silence. The breakdown of rapport. Isolation from each other. And finally, detachment and callousness about each other's feelings. A negative separation of the self from the marital arena.

This is alienation. It is critical to stem the tide before it reaches this point.

The most common denominator in fertility—a man's retreat and a woman's complicity in his retreat—endangers the relationship. When this happens, sooner or later most women come to the end of their rope. Sandra recognized that Tony was not ready to address the fertility problem. For a long time he saw it as her problem because his sperm were normal.

> I minded very much. In fact, he did not go to the doctor several times that I wanted him to. I asked him to go the first

> time, and he said no, he couldn't take off work, and I felt that he wasn't really there, emotionally. He wasn't ready for what was going on. I really wanted and needed the reassurance that he was there and involved. I felt like I was really going out on my limb, always doing it by myself. I would say, 'Come with me and talk to him.' 'No, I'm too busy.' So I was real sensitive and easily intimidated. I finally issued an ultimatum.

Sometimes so much stress is created by the polarization that puts the problem in a woman's lap that a couple considers separation. Sandra and Tony finally reached a crossroads in their relationship. She felt that the relationship had to change in order for it to continue. Having come to terms with her infertility, she was ready to move on with her life. She wanted to get legally married and adopt a child.

> I finally put it to Tony that it was important enough to me not to wait and I really wanted to get married and we had to make a decision, either get married or separate. So he decided he wanted to get married. That has given me a lot of reassurance and a lot of energy to pursue adoption. I felt like I was saying, 'You come with me this time. I want you to come and it's important.' And he's much more there.

In response to Sandra's determination to proceed to the next step in life, Tony examined the main issues in their relationship:

> There was a kind of reassessing of what was going on. We came to a point where we had to make a decision whether I was to leave and that was a big question in our relationship, whether we were really committed to each other.
>
> But I don't want to start a life with someone else. I feel committed to Sandra and our relationship. So that's part of our relationship—the infertility—and one of the things we need to go through and deal with as a couple.
>
> So there was a lot of deciding, 'how together are we?'

> We go through periods of being on each other's case, and that sort of thing. And I think a big issue was commitment.

EMOTIONAL NEGOTIATION

One way to undermine the polarization process—a way to short-circuit the entire problem and keep it on another level, out of the realm of fault and blame—is to take the whole issue and look at it as a series of negotiations in the relationship. Larry, in his search for a way to understand the dynamics between himself and Susan, had a sudden insight. He saw that their discussions about their fertility mirrored a process he was involved in in his daily work life. Whereas at work he was involved in the negotiation of commodities, at home he and Susan were involved in a long emotional negotiation.

> It's a negotiation, an emotional negotiation. I think people have trouble facing the feelings they have. It goes in cycles because the subject is so intense that only one person can bring it up at a time until it is sort of disarmed. And there are very rare times that you can really talk about it on the same honest level.
>
> In our experience, someone will take the lead, and someone will hang back. I mean, in general, Susan, you have been pushing, and it's taken a while to get me up to speed. Then once in a while we really get it right, and we have really good contact about it. Like the whole idea of adoption—it sort of peaks and flows. And that one has a lot of attributes of being an emotional negotiation.

As a professional negotiator, Larry was able to see the same dynamics at work in the relationship that he saw in his work life. Once he compared them and saw the similarities, Larry stopped taking negotiations with Susan personally.

> One of the things that is like a negotiation is that a lot of times you're more extreme than you really mean. You're testing out different things.

Looking upon their ongoing dialogue as an emotional negotiation enabled Larry to see the process free of its emotional overtones. Despite their many efforts to communicate clearly, Larry and Susan had been drifting toward polarization. The dynamics between them were defused when Larry stopped feeling as if he was somehow to blame. Instead of seeing himself as the unwitting villain who must have done something wrong—if only he knew what—he saw their dialogue as a tender process that had a life of its own, in the same way that his business negotiations did. When he stopped taking the effects of their infertility personally and let go of his efforts to distance himself, his entire attitude changed.

> I feel much more optimistic about our potential fertility than I ever did before. I feel like it's partially because of my involvement, feeling that I am now finally a part of this more than I have been for the three years when it was emotionally trying for Susan. All that time I felt that it was her problem and not my own. That's changed.

UNDOING DRIFT

When a man starts to look at himself more closely, his identity starts to change. He sees that his partner is right about something—this is a crisis. Men who discover they themselves have a fertility problem are forced to face their identity crisis sooner because of their own infertility. They no longer meet the central requirement for the stereotype of the real man. This discovery catapults a man into rethinking his identity, as it did for Matt.

JENNY: So I'm gung ho into the work-up. And I'm phoning around, talking to every adoption worker in five counties. And spending half my work life in the doctor's office. And I'm noticing, 'Hey, this is taking over my life, and what's the matter with him?'

MATT: I was feeling guilty. I was going through the machinations of, 'Would I be a good father? Would I not be a good father? Does my reluctance to go gung ho into this show mean that I want not to be a parent? Or that I don't want to be a secondhand parent, in the case of adoption?' You know, you get the message all through your life that the only way you can be a person and a family is to have children. So that is a big heavy trip. And I was battling with it. But not talking about it.

Sooner or later, a man redefines the problem. Regardless of whether or not he has a fertility factor. He agrees it is a mutual problem. Because the relationship is changing. And the loss of everything in life is threatening—everything that has to do with her and their life together. He wants to spend the rest of his life with her. And he does want a family. He wants to feel emotionally connected to her again. And he wants peace and order to return to their life. More than ever, he wants the problem solved. Right now. Who ever thought it would become such a big deal?

Women share these sentiments. As they recognize the threat that infertility poses to their relationship, they work to maintain their common bond with their partner. They struggle to stay objective. Despite the conflict that had developed in her relationship with Stan, Laura recognized the significance of his efforts:

When it's that time of the month, there have been several times when it was a perfect weekend to go bicycle touring with friends or up to the country. And he hasn't gone. And he hasn't made a fuss about it.

Everything he is doing, and he's doing a great deal—like wearing boxer shorts and making himself sexually

> available and not going in hot tubs—he's doing out of love. Because he's not an emotionally expressive person, so it's hard for me to sense how intense his love for me is. But I have really felt it through this experience because of all the sacrifices he is making.

WORKING TOGETHER

When a couple begins working together, they can stem the tide carrying them toward polarization. This is a turning point in the relationship.

After a long struggle over fertility that Theresa felt she carried on alone, she and Paul reached a turning point. Several things happened all at once. She had been protecting Paul—even from getting a semen analysis—until her physician insisted. The results showed that Paul had a low sperm count.

Meanwhile, she had reached her own turning point when she acknowledged to herself that she might never get pregnant. She began to take steps to deal more effectively with her fertility issues. Her determination to do more to help herself coincided with the report of the test results one week before a Resolve symposium.* To her surprise, Paul volunteered to go with her.

> Suddenly he got more involved. He was always interested. It was never like, 'It's your problem. I don't want to hear about it.' Or anything like that. But I was just so happy when he said, 'Oh, I'll go with you to the symposium.' It really meant a lot.
>
> He was glad he went. That was a real turning point. I think it was a first step in this whole new thing, looking back now.

---

*Resolve has sponsored over forty one-day conferences nationwide. Individual chapters of Resolve periodically sponsor conferences and workshops to disseminate information about infertility. Check with your local Resolve chapter or contact Resolve's national headquarters for more information.

Nevertheless, Theresa continued to worry about possible harm to their relationship:

> Right now he says he feels fine and that he can't worry about his infertility. So I hope what he is telling me he is feeling is what he is really feeling. I am concerned that there is more there. Maybe I'm not picking up on it or whatever . . .
>
> I say we have a pretty good marriage and I know him well. We try to be open but this is different. You are winging it. I just worry what he might be feeling and if it's pent up. I don't know, you don't know the right thing to do all the time.

Theresa and Paul began to work together to keep their infertility in perspective:

> When we were driving home from the symposium, he said, 'You could see couples there . . . I can imagine being married to someone who was more desperate to have children. We could propel that kind of anxiety. I could feel for people who were desperate.' And he spent a lot of time saying it can't obsess us.

Theresa described how this greater sense of togetherness had affected her:

> Things are bound to be better between two people if one is happier. I guess that's it—somehow, our relationship is better because I'm happier. That's probably the main effect. It's neat. I think if he hadn't gone to the seminar with me, hadn't become more involved in it, I would be almost embarrassed when it was my Resolve night. He is just not into that kind of thing. Now I come home and he wakes up and says, 'How was your meeting? What did you talk about?' Kind of recapping it. Almost every time I went he asked. It's not for him, but I think he saw the good in it, and why people would need it. When he thought it was my

> problem, I just had to worry about it by myself. He doesn't say any of that anymore.

Regardless of whether or not a man has a fertility problem himself, when he connects with his true self and acknowledges his fears, he gets involved. He realizes the problem is not going to go away without him.

A relationship is often in need of retuning at mid-life. It's not just fertility that raises questions, it's every interaction that goes amiss—the unclaimed baggage of a long-term relationship that must, at some point, be sorted, claimed, and acknowledged.

Once in touch with his feelings, a man may realize fertility is only one issue, and that the whole relationship needs his attention, like Greg did:

> Infertility was just a catalyst. Infertility did nothing but magnify some problems that we have had since the day we met. And the emotional side of my upbringing was pretty much limited, and I'm probably the most emotional one of my family.
>
> I felt like a cripple coming into infertility. So I wasn't prepared to deal with Gina's emotional outbursts. That's kind of a literary term for what they really were.
>
> I was waiting for the game to get over so we could get on with things. So pretty much I was sort of a blockhead emotionally and physically in helping out. That's what I brought to our little cauldron.

As he starts to change, he starts to show his "soft" side—that emotional, vulnerable, anxious side of himself. Which is what she really wants, anyway. What she needs. Company.

> Greg started attending some of my doctor appointments and began to see some of the emotional trauma. He began to understand it was a 'we' problem and not my problem, that it was an 'us' problem.
>
> —Gina

Greg described how his attitude changed from the time when he felt like the infertility work-up was proceeding without him and that there was little he could do about it:

> It's funny, because I'm the one who sits on the side. It's me who doesn't get the feeling of participation. Now I go to all Gina's exams—I try to stick around for all the procedures.
>
> There was a time when I didn't believe in taking aspirin, whether she was taking it or I was taking it. But—we are together. It's my problem and Gina's problem. It's a couple problem. I don't see it as her problem. It is not male-related, as far as we know. But it's still our problem. For me to stand outside or to stay at home, that isn't going to help. For me to stay in the dark emotionally and intellectually isn't going to help our problem.

Once partners are talking with each other about their infertility and feel they are working together, problems that appear to be intractable can be aired and discussed. Discussing when to stop medical treatment, Greg said to Gina:

> You haven't hit the wall yet. I've hit it a couple of times. I've hit my limits technologically, and only my backing off a little bit and trying to look beyond kept me going. The third miscarriage was one and the GNRH-A stuff was the other.* I'm not the greatest advocate of experimental medicine. After your third miscarriage, when you said, 'Well, I think I could put up with at least two more,' I just thought, 'Two more you can put up with?' Wondering what sack you were going to be carrying me in at that point. Two more miscarriages. Geez. Give me a break.

No longer needing to defend her position because she had received so much support from Greg, Gina was able to drop her militant stand and say, "I know, it was a stupid thing to say."

---

*GNRH-A is a pituitary hormone-like substance used during ovarian stimulation in in vitro fertilization and related technologies.

Once a man and a woman have begun to meet each other, the sense of being polar opposites—of working at cross-purposes—begins to fade. They unite in their efforts. Each of them stops feeling so vulnerable, so lost. The child in each of them recedes into the background as the threat to their relationship wanes. In a discussion of his relationship with Gina, Greg concluded:

> Throughout our marriage and relationship I don't think we have been the greatest delvers into our heart of hearts and we don't exchange those most intimate of confidences easily. With a year of therapy, we still don't really know all the answers.

All these identity changes don't mean the relationship returns to where it was before. Now that they have found out they are separate from each other—different as individuals, as men and women—it raises a whole new realm of possibilities for a couple. Especially since the future is still unknown.

Paula and Lou reflected on the effect infertility has had on their relationship.

> PAULA: I think it has done different things. Sometimes it has made us a lot closer; sometimes it hasn't. . . . It created real barriers. But it shifts, you know.

> LOU: You can't point to it as doing either positive or negative things. I think in any relationship that is healthy, it changes and continues to change. So from that standpoint this has not been major. It has not been more major than a lot of other things that have happened along the way. I could name several.

CHAPTER 11

GETTING HELP

People need support. They need other people. Humans are the only species that cannot survive without meaningful human contact—touch, care, communication. But when a couple has a fertility problem, they can't get their needs met by each other alone. In fact, no one can. It's unreasonable to expect a partner to meet all of one's needs at *any* time in life. But if they can't turn to each other at this particular time, each partner feels really alone.

When efforts to cope—with the relationship, with infertility, with the rest of the world—are not working, it's a good idea to seek help. It has been found in clinical practice as well as in the research for this book that getting outside help is one of the single most effective steps a couple can take to deal with infertility.

But couples hesitate to take this step. Why is this? There are many reasons. If you have been contemplating turning to a support group or to a professional but get cold feet every time you seriously consider it, you will probably find your doubts described here. The reasons people balk at getting help are based, for the most part, on their fears of what will happen if they do. Will it make matters worse?

Getting help is an acknowledgment that something is wrong. And who wants to admit that? It smacks of failure. Keeping up a solid front in the face of desperation, Stan said of his relationship with Laura,

> I would get counseling if our relationship was in trouble. But it's not. We don't have a problem.

Men and women may think, "I should be able to do this on my own, and if I can't, there is something wrong with me." They worry that they will find out the worst about themselves. They may fear what they will find if they plumb their unknown depths. They equate seeking help with self-exposure, even though they are not sure what will be exposed. Whatever it turns out to be may be too terrible to face. And if *they* can't face it, how will their partner respond?

Greg and Gina analyzed the barriers with which they had started therapy:

> GREG: You don't talk to anybody in my family if you have problems. Neither one of us grew up with the frame of mind of 'When you have a problem, go talk to a third party.'
>
> GINA: Both Greg and I come from backgrounds that said, 'If you have to go to a shrink, you are nuts.' Greg's way was gunnysack it all, or you play like you don't have problems, period. Mine was internalizing it all and eat yourself alive. That's how you cope. Therapy has been a very enlightening and empowering experience for me.

Men and women worry about their relationship. How will it weather this self-exposure in front of other people? They're afraid of what bright lights will do to the fabric of the relationship. Can it handle the strain? They don't want others to see them fight. They don't want to look too closely at some of their other interchanges. They're not sure they handled that last one well. What if their deepest fears are true? What if their fertility problem is a sign they aren't compatible? Whatever they do, they don't want to make things worse than they are, so they protect the relationship, as Theresa did:

> We don't have a problem communicating with each other. I don't think we do, anyway. We decided not to go to those marriage workshops because we don't want to make a problem where we don't have one.

This set of fears—that we aren't as together as we think we are, that the worst about us will become known, that we are somehow terrible, that we should not be together—is widespread. Most people—not just people who have a fertility problem—carry these fears buried deep inside themselves.

But they *are* fears—they are not truths. What *is* the truth?

The truth is, turning to outside help is a reflection of strength, not weakness. What happens when we take this step? We learn about our strengths. As individuals. As a couple. We learn to understand our fears. We learn that the bogeyman standing in the shadows—that terrible person we think we might be—isn't really there, he's just in our imagination.

When women and men begin to let go of their fears about themselves and the relationship, it frees them to start communicating more effectively with each other. It frees them to ask themselves how they *really* think and feel about something, instead of taking their traditional stance or course of action. It enables them to start exploring their universe again—together—as they did when they first met. The big difference this time is that now they recognize they are two individuals, with perspectives that are often different, not two parts of a symbiotic whole. Being different from each other makes life together interesting, vital.

A couple's identification with each other, which may have taken a beating in the search for fertility, is renewed. And given a chance to grow. When men and women are united in their efforts, the meaning of their partnership is reinforced.

What triggers people to seek help? The threat partners feel to their relationship is a major incentive. Gina and Greg described how this came about:

> GINA: Our doctor looked at us one day and said, 'How are you doing?' I started crying. We figured it was definitely time to do something.

> GREG: He introduced us to a therapist and Gina started going, and then I was asked to come along. I treated that experience much like I would going to any doctor's office. It was the last thing on my mind I wanted to do, but after a little more enlightenment on my part, I got into the swing of

> what we were trying to accomplish there. After a year of work with her I grew up a little bit and Gina and I learned to, if not talk openly, at least grunt meaningful noises at each other. There are still some things to work out.

A second reason for not seeking help is specific to men. Men are trying to live up to the stereotype of the *real* man. They are supposed to be strong. They are not supposed to have needs, or show signs of being soft. And they are not supposed to have failures. So if they equate going to a group or seeking counseling as a sign of failure, they won't want to do it. A man may see it as a statement about himself, that he is a failure as a person, to have to resort to such measures. Worse still, if he starts owning up to all his fears, maybe the worst *will* happen—he will dissolve in a puddle of tears.

Not only that, men may find it hard to talk about their feelings, to express their emotions. And if so, the whole endeavor may be a threat. A man may feel that his partner can talk circles around him in expressing her feelings and making her needs known. When she looks inside herself, it may seem to him that she comes up with these profound, even brilliant, analyses of why she feels what she feels and what it means. Something he would never have thought of. It makes him feel dumb. He may reason that if he goes with her to a group or a counselor, she will be articulate and he will seem like a clod who can't think straight, who says the wrong things.

These are fears, not reality. Sometimes these fears are only overcome by a greater fear—of losing the relationship. The fear of this ultimate loss motivated Greg:

> Gina, fortunately, got unhappy enough that she did something about it. And then I guess I was scared enough of losing the relationship that I was willing to go into therapy. I used to think of every way I could avoid it, hoping that in six weeks Gina would solve her problems and we could get on with our lives.

What *is* real? Women don't want men to be strong and impassive. They want men to express themselves. They want to be in contact with the *real* person, not with the stereotype for a real man. A woman recognizes she may be in the crisis of her life. She wants company. Togetherness.

Not only that, if a woman spends more time on introspection than her partner does, she knows it. It doesn't mean she expects him to automatically come up to speed with her on the subject of fertility or on any other subject that may arise. She just wants him to try to work with her on their issues, whatever those issues are. If he can start by saying what is on his mind, that's enough. It's a start. Whatever else comes after that will unfold, depending on the couple and the route they take. And by that time they will be reconnected to each other. Their sense of isolation will have faded.

What other truths can I tell you about seeking help? The truth is, there will be moments of pain. And yes, sometimes the pain may be intense. But this is a small price to pay for the pleasure of rediscovering each other, for the excitement of discovering oneself. Examining your feelings and exploring yourselves with each other is not only the main task on the road to resolution, it's essential to effectively begin the next stage of life.

And there is a bonus: You gain the potential to enrich your relationship with each other. And to strengthen your relationship with your self. Greg described what happened to him in therapy:

> I entered therapy and played wrestling matches with the therapist. I began to slowly break down and acknowledge that there are a lot of things that made me very, very unhappy and were totally unrelated to Gina and her emotional interpretation of the world. Basically, I was handed a bill of goods when I was just a wee embryo and repackaged and relabeled in that same packing material for my whole life. In therapy it just kind of sloughed off and got turned around and looked at and repackaged. Now *I'm* doing the packaging.
>
> Therapy was a wonderful experience. I couldn't have done it without infertility.

A CHECKLIST FOR SEEKING HELP

Here is my list of recommendations. Keeping them in mind, think about the danger signals I have described in relationships. Consider what the people in this book have said about grief and loss. About identity. About unity. Ask yourself if any of this applies to you. If fertility is an issue for you or for the person you love, it would be some kind of miracle to avoid all the potential pitfalls you face. So if you have identified even one issue I have raised, consider seeking help. Believe me, life will get better.

1. Don't wait. The earlier help is sought, the better. When time passes, feelings that have no outlet build up and become explosive.
2. Talk with each other about it. If you have doubts about turning to outside help, discussing your concerns with your partner will help you to talk about the *real* issue: how fertility issues are affecting each of you and your relationship.
3. Explore the possible resources. There are various kinds of help available, from small groups run by Resolve to individual psychotherapy and couples counseling. Find out what's available in your area, then think about what you would be most comfortable with. In the pages ahead I describe different couples' experiences with different modes. Use these comments to help you clarify what would work best for you. For example, have you used any of these techniques before? If you have, whatever you did in the past may be most comfortable for you to try first, whether it is to join a group or to seek a counselor alone. If you have never tried any of these kinds of help, you may feel most at ease in a group, initially. You can just sit there and observe, joining in at your own pace.

4. Consider your own gender issues. I have talked continuously in this book about the differences between men and women. Consider what the issues are for you in seeking help. For example, if you are a woman considering psychotherapy, would talking to another woman be especially helpful? If so, does her parenting potential or personal experience matter? Use your answers to guide you in selecting someone.

   Or, if you are a man who has gone to a Resolve group with your partner only to find that you are the only man there, are you comfortable with that? Would you be more at home in a group that has men in it? Group makeup varies. If you're ill at ease, don't give up. Keep searching until you find the right group.
5. What can you afford? The cost of seeking help is a major consideration for couples whose budget may already be strained by paying for infertility treatment. The various possibilities range from modest fees for Resolve groups to a more substantial output of funds for couples counseling and individual psychotherapy. So money is an important consideration. But try not to use it as an excuse to do nothing. It may be more vital to your health and the health of your relationship than the medical treatment you or your partner receives. It depends on the couple.
6. How long will it take? That all depends on you, and on the type of help you opt for. Resolve support groups are generally eight weeks long. If they continue, that is negotiated within the group itself. Other groups may be available with different formats, sponsored by hospitals, community agencies, or individual counselors or therapists. Ask the professionals you know who provide other infertility services for suggestions.

Counseling or psychotherapy may be short-term or long-term, lasting from a few months to over a year. It is up to you. You may want to start and see how it goes. You can stop when you want to.

You can try out several different counselors or several different modalities before deciding. It is perfectly okay to do this. The whole purpose of getting help is to make life better for you and your partner. You hold the reins.

There is one form of counseling and psychotherapy I hope you won't need to use. It's called crisis intervention. It is done on a short-term basis with people who are in an intense crisis. People whose world has completely collapsed around them. Don't wait until it comes to this:

> After my last IVF cycle I was supposed to go back to work.* But I didn't have any energy. I was feeling terribly depressed. I decided I'd better see a therapist. My husband was already in therapy. The therapist wondered why I hadn't been in therapy before. I just thought I was handling it well enough. I don't know—somehow it seemed like I was weathering it pretty well and I . . . well, I knew I was depressed but I thought that was a normal reaction for what I'm struggling with, so I would just live with it and hopefully, when things got ironed out, it would clear up. I think that wasn't good foresight because of the cumulative effect of all this. I can hardly get through the day. And I've been on leave for two months now so pretty soon I have to go back to work. I don't know how I will do it. My husband is at the end of his rope.
>
> —Lisa

Or to this:

> We've been screaming at each other a lot. It has just been a real difficult time for us. Talking to another person is sort of a vacation from it. We don't have to deal with each other for once. There's a lot of tension between us now. If we didn't have a strong marriage, after this thing with my career and

*In vitro fertilization (IVF) is often the last step in infertility treatment. An expensive and complex medical process, it is emotionally intense, and persons who undergo it may experience depression and emotional exhaustion if an IVF cycle does not conclude in a pregnancy.

> the DI charade we went through, not many relationships could go through this.
>
> —Jerry

RESOLVE SUPPORT GROUPS

When dealing with infertility alone becomes too stressful, couples often turn first to a Resolve support group.* Women usually initiate this kind of involvement, as Angie did:

> ANGIE: I heard about Resolve's support groups, and I was sure it would help us, so I just told Rick we should go. We had gone to a self-help group before, and that was a good experience.
>
> RICK: So at first I was going, but without any enthusiasm.
>
> ANGIE: Just sort of perfunctorily, right?
>
> RICK: There weren't that many other men there. And that bothered me. But as we've gone along, my commitment to going to those meetings increased.

Laura was adamant about the importance of joining a group. She thought she would have a fight on her hands, getting Stan to agree to go. He surprised her.

> That's why I dragged us, insisted that we join the Resolve group. Because I knew there would be some kind of support there, a different kind of support from what I would like to get from Stan. I just couldn't go it alone.
>
> It turned out he was more than willing to go because he

*For information about Resolve support groups in your area, contact your local Resolve chapter.

> wanted to find out what he suspected, which was that other men were going through the same things he was, you know, with sex, and our communication problems and all that. He found that out. He feels really positive about the group. In fact, a couple of times I was sick, and he went without me. There was no question that he wasn't going to go. He just got ready to go and he went.

But sometimes men are reluctant to join a support group. Sometimes women go by themselves when their husbands do not want to be involved, as Theresa did:

> It ended up being pretty small. It was all women. The first meeting there were about seven women and one husband came. He was a nice man, and he shared his feelings, but he didn't come back. I could see that he felt funny, being the only man there. It was tough on him.

Sometimes men agree to attend a group when infertility is compounded by another crisis. Ron had not wanted to attend a group. When he simultaneously learned of his infertility and lost his job, he changed his mind, to Celia's relief:

> Ron wasn't terribly in favor of a Resolve group. I guess it's like anything else—people have to hit rock bottom. There has to be a crisis and that has to be the motivator.
>
> I had been harping all this time about Resolve and he didn't listen to me. But after that he was the one who called Resolve to find out about groups.

Celia found that attending a group dramatically affected how she and Ron dealt with their infertility. On her first visit, Celia realized she was carrying attitudes around with her about being abnormal. These began to dissipate when she met other group members:

> When I went to the first group one of my first thoughts was, 'Well, gee, everyone here looks so normal.'

Attending a group helped Celia and Ron put their infertility in perspective.

> Ron says one thing about going to the group is you realize that everybody's problems are worse than yours are. I mean, medically we had the simplest problem in the group.
>
> In a peer support group you are with people like you who are in the same boat and you get started talking about your problems. I have to say the Resolve group was an equal, if not more important part, than each of us being in therapy. It really was a catalyst for us.

The group helped them talk to each other:

> The group was very powerful for both of us. It helped us talk. What we couldn't say to each other at home, we could say to each other in the group.

Resolve support groups may be a good source of information as well as support:

> When you're an infertile couple, you don't just rely on what a doctor tells you, you try to find out as much as possible other ways, like getting involved with Resolve. That's been the most uplifting thing about Resolve—the exchange of information. It's been fabulous.
>
> —Carrie

> The week before I had the laparoscopy I told everyone in our support group. It was probably the second week we met. Our support group was full of people who were pretty far along. So most of them had had the experience and they described it to me. I hadn't heard anything my doctor said, so that helped a lot.
>
> —Betsy

The hard part of a Resolve support group may come when it ends, if some people end up with babies and others do not:

> We met for a long time. It must have been at least six months. The last two social events after we stopped meeting just didn't click, though, partly because all but two couples had babies and it was hard on the two that didn't. And on the others that did.
>
> —Celia

Theresa summed up the main purpose of a Resolve support group when she said:

> I really believe in the benefit of communication, and the therapy that goes with it. And that's what led me to sign up for the support group. I think I get a lot of emotional support there.

SEEKING COUNSELING OR THERAPY

Couples often enter counseling together because they feel overwhelmed by the combination of infertility and other problems in their lives. Life had been turbulent for Betsy and Jonathan during their infertility treatment.

> BETSY: Our lives have not been easy. Jonathan's father died last fall. Then this spring Jonathan lost his job in a very traumatic way. He was fired, and it was completely unfair. And I got into a very bad job situation. I now have another terrible job.
>
> JONATHAN: And your mother was in the hospital with cancer.
>
> BETSY: Yes, she's really acute right now. Anyway, the last year has been a traumatic year. It would be a traumatic year in anyone's life, and it was.
>
> JONATHAN: Remember? You wanted to get out of town and move to Oregon.

> BETSY: Yeah, life just seemed horrible at that time. It was very awful.

Their solution was to seek help. Betsy said,

> Jonathan, wasn't it last fall that we started seeing the counselor? It was around that time—when you were out of work for a while. We went to a marriage counselor. It was not a good time in our lives. We . . . it was the worst time in our relationship.
>
> We started seeing a marriage counselor and were doing much better together. Things got better, and it was really nice again. I can't say all our problems were infertility because they weren't. But it didn't help.
>
> Medical treatment was additional stress that we couldn't deal with. Thank God it became more important to make sure our marriage and our life was all right instead of going to some doctor. It really is up to us, anyway.

Women and men seek counseling or therapy for a variety of reasons. Some seek individual therapy. Laura was planning to go into counseling to help her to grieve.

> I'm absolutely convinced that I really must get counseling and I'm holding off until I start this hMG business. I'm just terrified, terrified at the possibility that that's the ultimate failure. There's nothing beyond it, there's no hope beyond that. And I really want somebody to be there for me and help me work through my grief.

Celia sought therapy because of marital problems.

> The reason I went into therapy to begin with was that our marriage was on the rocks. Not because of infertility.

It is important to choose the right counselor or therapist. The central concern that everyone has is the counselor's ability to relate to the experience of infertility:

> I am very lucky. It was just a coincidence, but it took my therapist eighteen months to conceive, so she had been through it. She had experienced infertility.
>
> —Celia

> When I asked my doctor for a referral, he gave me the name of a therapist who had been through infertility. But she was just too far away. I didn't have the energy to drive that far. So I chose somebody I knew slightly. I knew she had been pregnant. I thought, 'This is someone who, if she has a child, can't underestimate how important this is to me.' I think someone who would choose not to be pregnant may not understand my feelings. And I feel comfortable talking to her.
>
> —Lisa

Couples often weigh what will work best for them, counseling or a support group. Matt explained how they made the decision:

> We never went to a Resolve group. I didn't want to because I thought, 'I don't want to sit around with a bunch of people and complain. Or find out about other people's failures. I have enough problems of my own, and I don't want to have to take the burden of someone else's failures and help them through it. Here I am helping me and her through our own problems.' It just didn't appeal to us at all. We went to couples counseling instead.

While women may find counseling with another woman especially helpful during infertility, men may feel that they need to talk with another man, as Matt did:

> MATT: I never saw our counselor by myself. A woman is not going to know how I feel. I just didn't feel that there was someone who would know how I felt. Even though she might have an infertility problem herself, it's not the same thing. It's like me counseling somebody about being preg-

nant. I have no idea what they are talking about. I don't know what the feelings are, I don't know what any of it is about. So I didn't pursue it. I really don't know what is available for men.

JENNY: Men don't go to counseling.

MATT: No, men don't go to counseling. It is very difficult for me to talk to a counselor. I went once to this guy. But I have no communication with him. I think he's a jerk.

As women and men move through different stages in addressing their fertility, their needs may change. Jenny's did:

I was in counseling with someone who is a Supermom. If I were going to do counseling now, I would want to talk to somebody who can be a role model for a full life without children.

Gina and Greg talked about how the decision to seek counseling came about:

GINA: Our doctor makes a real big deal out of getting help. Part of his work-up generally is a discussion of this. He thinks this is real important and he highly recommends it. The gist of it was that he didn't know too many people who could get through this without some kind of counseling or therapy. It is pretty astounding for anybody in the medical community to say, 'I can only deal with part of this problem. You really need to go get some help.' That in itself is fairly revolutionary, which is another reason why we did it.

It was other problems emphasized by the infertility that got us in there and we probably spent three quarters of that year talking about things unrelated to infertility and finally got around to the infertility. Not necessarily in that order, not necessarily that clean-cut. I'm sure that isn't particularly unusual, either. Infertility is a super-stress on top of every-

> thing else that just makes some of it—more sort of foundation problems—look worse or be more uncomfortable.

When women and men near the end of the infertility work-up, they often view counseling differently than they previously had:

> GINA: We terminated with the option of returning. In the beginning she had said that this is not a long-term situation in her experience. I don't know if she gave us an end-time, like a year or year and a half, but it wasn't a surprise to any of us that this was about to happen. We felt like it was time.

> GREG: We stopped once, then went back, then stopped again. We can perform on the wire as long as we know she's down there. She's our safety net.

> GINA: I don't see how anybody goes through this process without getting some therapy. I really don't. I don't know how people survive it. When you sit down in a Resolve group and you see these couples looking at each other like the other one is out of their ever lovin' mind, when they openly admit clearly that people aren't communicating their needs . . . I really don't know.

Counseling can be a potent ingredient in the process of resolution.

CHAPTER 12

CHANGES

The woman who had ushered me in was sitting on her couch, talking composedly. Her dark brown hair hung in soft curls around her face. She sat there, straight-backed, in a dress of soft shades of blue that reflected the blue of her eyes. She wore new high heels, planted firmly on the carpet. This woman seemed to radiate quiet strength. Hands folded in her lap, she talked quietly, but with feeling, about her failed hopes, her altered dreams. She talked about quirks of fate, and about loss. She talked about realizations about her husband, and about herself. About growing up in poverty, and about settling for less. About the future, and about change.

I felt as if I had never seen this woman before.

The last time I visited this neighborhood, I came to this house. I walked past the children playing on the sidewalk, past the grassy plots of green, past the pine tree, to this door. The woman who answered the door that day bore little resemblance to this woman. There was some similarity in her angular jaw, the color of her eyes. But that woman could hardly be this woman. She wore a nondescript housedress. Her hair was permed in tight little curls reminiscent of another age. She sat on her couch slumped forward, staring at the floor, answering my questions in terse little sentences, often breaking into tears, and looking away.

That day her pain was so raw and her grief so great that the sound of her own voice seemed intolerable to her. She was in a paroxysm of pain, a torment so huge it seemed violent to intervene with words, with questions. People usually seem to find relief in talking to me after the first few minutes. But talking with her never got easy. She was in too much pain.

I finally felt that there was nothing to be done but to acknowledge her pain with silence. So we sat there together silently. Then I touched her on the arm and left.

This is Marilyn. This *is* the same woman. And yet she's not the same.

On the first visit, Marilyn's pain had been so acute, her grief so intense, that I wondered what could be done to help her get through this time. What could I say? I had suggested the possibility of adoption, the importance of finding other ways of including children in her life. I recommended counseling. I had urged her to try to talk more with her partner. I recommended that she confide in her friends, that she seek out her pastor at church. But, having made these suggestions, I concluded that there was little more that could be done. Whatever she did was up to her.

Three months after the first visit, Marilyn had become a different person.

> Right after I saw you, I lost my job. Since then I have felt terrible about myself. They didn't believe I was going to the doctor all that time. We came to a mutual agreement it was best to part. Finally, they agreed that if I would quit, they wouldn't fire me. And the irony of it—I prided myself on my work!
>
> So I signed up for the fall semester at the college. I'm full time in this program, but I honestly don't know if I'm interested. I just had to do something. Anything. I can't go on like this.

Marilyn had been in an infertility work-up off and on since she was 30. She had tried everything, and now she was applying for an in vitro fertilization program (IVF), a program she could not afford.

> Now I'm 35. I feel really old. I'm really angry about the infertility. I feel like I'm not grown up, somehow. Children make you feel mature. I work with all these other women who are in their late forties, early fifties. And their kids are

almost grown. They treat me like I'm a child, like I'm not an adult. That's why I went out and bought myself some new clothes. I thought, 'I'm not a girl anymore. I'm a woman. I better start looking like one.'

Marilyn was raised in a strict religious environment, where children were seen but not heard. And they were poor. Her childhood affected how she saw her life stretching out ahead of her.

I grew up out in the country, and my mother was old. So I always wanted to have children before I got too old. My parents were always too tired to go to PTA meetings. And I had to always be quiet. They were always after me not to make any noise. My mother was very strict. She raised me the way she was raised herself. She doesn't believe you should talk about your feelings or about your problems.

There was a lot of poverty. So they didn't have any expectations for me. Because I was a girl, they thought I would get married and have children.

She thought so herself.

My church was always pushing having children. I grew up thinking that's what would happen. I spent all this time just sort of waiting. First I was waiting to meet someone. I went to work after high school, and I took a few college courses. But mainly I worked. Then I met my husband when I was 22. He was the first man I ever dated. We got married when I was 24. When the opportunity to marry came up, I was desperate to leave home, so I married.

But he wasn't ready to have children. I worked so he could finish college. And then he got a job offer in another part of the country. I followed him from one place to another, just working and waiting.

I spent all this time just sort of waiting. Waiting for my husband. Waiting to get pregnant. And now I feel like I don't

> have anything—I don't have an education. I always thought, 'I'll take any job, because soon I'll be pregnant.' I still don't want to adopt. What if they leave you when they are 19?

When she turned 28, she got tired of waiting for life to start.

> I didn't have a good understanding of what was happening to me, then. I don't know . . . All of a sudden I was 28 and I wanted to date. And getting married—I wished that I didn't get married so soon. I didn't know anything about men. I didn't know what I wanted. But I don't know now whether I would have found other romances, or what.
>
> I wondered what it would have been like to date other men. To marry other men. I had second thoughts about the marriage. But after a while they subsided.
>
> But now, I don't know . . . I can't talk to him. It's not deep.

At 35, Marilyn is finally waking up. And taking action to change her life.

> I feel like life has passed me by. I never had a well-formed idea of what I would do in life. Except have children and raise a family. And that hasn't happened. I was lulled into thinking it would happen. Then time started passing, faster and faster. And we lived this nomadic existence, and I have never made friends that fast, anyway. So I had no one to talk to about it.
>
> When I lost my job, I had to do something. So I went to a counselor. And that has helped.
>
> And I have started to change my life. I am going to start teaching Sunday School again. I need to be around children.

Six months passed. On my third visit, the children that used to play on Marilyn's lawn were playing in her house. And she was still working on her college degree, and planning to adopt.

Once our identity starts to change, everything else in life is altered. Forever. The world becomes a different place. Or do we see differences where none exist? Is it only that *we* are different? That *we* have changed? How we think and what we think about is no longer the same. We see the past in a new light. We see those around us with fresh eyes. We look more closely at everything about ourselves—how we spend our time, the work we do, the relationship with our partner. We reformulate every aspect of our lives.

When things don't go according to plan, we question what life is all about. Where do we fit into this giant scheme? Why didn't it happen like it was supposed to? Eventually, we ask ourselves if we still want what we wanted when we started out. Sometimes the answer is yes, and sometimes it's no. But once we begin asking ourselves these questions, we start examining the whole complex mosaic called life.

As we begin this odyssey of self-examination, we reconstruct our history. We rewrite our life script so that it flows along in some meaningful way. We identify the crossroads. We mark the significant events.

Each of us has a life history that is unique. A story that is idiosyncratic, that changes as we change. A life in the here-and-now that transforms itself as our culture changes, as well as a life in the past that we interpret and recast as we age. When we start to rethink our life, certain events in the past take on new meaning. These events become symbols—ways of interpreting what has happened to us. These symbols make sense out of the nonsensical, the unpredictable, the unexpected.

One day I was visiting Jeff at his home. He lives in a striking house he built himself—he is a contractor. I was there to learn his life history—his story of all the events that led up to the present.

> I grew up in a greenhouse. My family farmed for a living. My parents didn't get along. There was a lot of fighting. Our house was right next to the the fields. So I spent all my time out there in the fields. Out there I was free—no one telling

> me what to do. It was quiet out there. I used to lie on my back and stare up at the sky, and daydream.

Suddenly, I became more aware of my surroundings. I looked up and up—into space. I looked around, and there was glass everywhere. This house was one huge room without walls. I was sitting in a giant, modernistic version of a greenhouse, full of space and light.

Jeff's house is a symbol—of overcoming the conflicts of the past. His self-determination is embodied in a new greenhouse, one of his own making.

It is not just events themselves that become symbols. It is what we do with them. How we view ourselves in relation to them. How we used them in the past, and how we use them now, to make sense of our world.

Jeff described the push-pull dynamics in his family—his feeling of rejection that alternated with feeling engulfed. He talked about how he finally severed the family knot to live out his symbol of freedom—building houses.

> When I was 16, my parents thought the town was so small that I would get a lousy education, so they sent me to live with an aunt in another state. I spent two years there.
>
> When I was away, they moved, and they didn't even tell me they moved until I called them up for the holiday season. I was going to get the train home, and my parents said, 'No, don't do that, we have moved.' And I said, 'But all my friends are there. How could you do that without asking me? Without telling me?' And their response was, 'You're off with Aunt Mae. What the hell do you care?'
>
> When I came back after two years, I found out that I couldn't live with my parents any longer. I'd gotten used to being on my own, and they couldn't understand it. We had a series of big arguments and fights, and I finally just left home one night, and let them know a week later that I was still alive.

> It changed our relationship. But it took physically walking out the door to do it. And every time I said I was going to do it, my mother would run up to the door and throw her arms up and say, 'Go ahead, break your dad's heart.' So finally I said, 'Shit, it's breaking *my* heart. I'm leaving.' And I left. I went to a big city and worked.
>
> I haven't gone back much. I've been involved in my own life. I love what I do. I love building houses.

These symbols are the threads of our lives that enable us to link past with present. No matter how impossible an event initially seems to be, no matter how chaotic life seemed last month, or last year, sooner or later we find the recognizable threads that hold some meaning. We begin knitting them together into a new fabric. When we begin to do this, we have begun to reconstruct our life, to weave a biography that is uniquely our own.

Carrie linked her past with her present by asking herself what she could compare with her infertility. What else had happened to her that was unexpected? That had required all her strength? And she asked herself, What had she done with those experiences? How had she coped? How could those experiences in the past help her to deal with her infertility now?

> History is important when you're looking back on how your life has evolved. It's also important in trying to predict the future. But you can't let it overwhelm you. You can't let things you can't achieve do you in. Childbearing, birth, pregnancy is something I can't achieve. I shouldn't consider myself a failure because I have a lot of other options in what I can do.
>
> I do think you are shaped by your experiences, and my experience has been having to rebound to survive. I do see myself as a survivor. I think about my experiences and traumas and bad experiences—a lot of complicated experiences—and I always come back from them. I think I will apply that to the situation. I am already doing that now

because I am removing myself more and more from the fact of infertility ruling my life. It's a complex phasing out.

And the longer I go through it, the more I phase it out. I used to get uptight about it but now it's almost like dealing with my father's death. It happened, I didn't understand it, but I've phased it out. It was a moment in my life, and it affected me. But it's affected me because I have looked back on those experiences. I don't know exactly how it affected me, except that it made me independent.

I just don't let certain things eat away at me. There are usually really trivial things I tend to focus on. The traumas in my life, I don't. I have dealt with a lot. I could have let that sexual abuse in my childhood ruin me. It could have really screwed me up. But I haven't let it. I reflect on it. It happened. I learned from it. I can't say that learning was a positive experience. But you have to move on, you have to say, 'That happened.' And you go on. It's history.

THE SEARCH FOR SELF-CONSISTENCY

After a period of inner chaos, we automatically begin to integrate past and present. The self requires a sense of consistency. Too much inconsistency—too much internal chaos—leads to feeling permanently off-center. If feeling off-center persists too long—for years on end—a person decompensates and becomes less functional.

The struggle for self-consistency goes on through life, never ending. Our faith in ourselves and our hopes for the future are grounded in this sense of continuity. Continuity is *the* issue of mid-life, as we search for the meaning in our lives. No matter what our set of life circumstances is, we are faced with the same set of questions: "Who am I?" and "What is the meaning of my life?" We find that we are holding a collection of the different parts of ourself, pieces that don't necessarily match up to who we are in the world. These definitions of ourselves that we have held at the various stages of our life are sometimes at odds with each other. And often they are at odds with the person we see when we step outside ourself for a more objective look.

Suddenly it may seem that nothing fits together the way we thought it would. Instead of an easy linear path along life's stages, we find ourselves holding a crazy quilt—a jigsaw puzzle of the many pieces that make us up—and they don't fit together very well. There are some pieces missing. And sometimes pieces overlap, or don't fit right. There's no synthesis, no cohesion. At least we can no longer see it, or feel it.

> There is this total suspension, an isolation from normal life processes—social, cultural, physical processes—that 95 percent of our population takes for granted. The things that make up the life and breath of our society. And all of a sudden our breath is choked off and we are sitting quietly, choking.
>
> It sure makes you think about what you took for granted, almost the mindlessness of it, marching from cradle to grave, following the recess bell. Then all of a sudden, you're standing outside the schoolyard, looking in and not being a part of it.
>
> —Gina

We feel lost. We were anchored to our universe, and now we have been cast adrift. We grope around, trying to collect the pieces, frantically trying to fit them back into place. But they no longer fit. Things that made sense last year suddenly have no rhyme or reason. In an effort to find the puzzle's key, we go back to the beginning. Back to who our parents wanted us to be. Then we look at who *we* wanted to be. Then we come to a third thing: who we are. And who we are is usually different from who our parents wanted us to be *or* who we thought we would become.

> As a woman I get so upset over the societal conditioning that you have to be a wife, you have to be a mother. There are all

> these have-tos. There are days when I ask, 'Why do I want this?' Am I that badly keyed into societal conditioning? I can't answer that question. It is one of the nightmares of my life.
>
> On one level you struggle so hard for what is personally intimate, which is the relationship that you have and what you want that relationship to bear. And on another hand, it's being knowledgeable of society and its pressures and maneuverings. Is that because of the kind of work I do? Are we going through this hell because I can't meet society's expectations for women? Give me a break.
>
> —Gina

Thinking about who we are isn't so simple. Because the more we think about it, the less certain we may be that we know who we are. And then we start asking ourselves, "Who am I?" all over again.

> I sacrificed part of myself in the infertility struggle. Somewhere along the line I lost 'me' a lot. Regardless of whether I get pregnant or not, that is the problem I need to work on, even if I get pregnant tomorrow, you know—'Okay, now you are pregnant.' I don't just want to be a pregnant woman or a mother. There is still 'me.'
>
> So that is the main thing I am getting out of this experience. That's good.
>
> —Theresa

It is the discontinuities in life that lead us to go on searching for the continuity in ourself. So when fertility becomes an issue as we enter mid-life, this inner search becomes acute, as the different parts of our life seem particularly unrelated to each other. In the process, we may get a little lost—disoriented—about who we are.

We are looking beyond sheer survival of this experience to its potential for personal growth. Depending on which leg of this journey you are on, you may feel this is an impossible goal—that right now you just want to get through the day. But getting through the day is not equivalent to our need as humans to have a purpose in life, to find outlets for the realization of our generative potential. Finding meaning in life is a necessity that we strive toward no matter how difficult our personal path may be. It is what differentiates us from other species—the ability to create symbols from which we gain sustenance.

This ability to nurture oneself through abstract ideas—through a future we construct for ourselves—is the essence of being a person. This inner striving may seem to be dormant in you for the time being, while you deal with daily life. But sooner or later you will again experience it as a need, just as vital as food and sleep. It is what gives us our humanity.

CONSTRUCTING THE LIFE STORY

When we reach a crossroads in life and are uncertain about the direction we should take, our own life story may help to guide us. As we rethink our identity, we pick and choose from the entire history of our life to develop the themes in our life story. This is not necessarily a conscious, intentional process. It involves our feelings, our senses, our intuition. Our story is whatever makes sense to us as an explanation of who we are. It develops in little spurts—driving on the freeway, walking in the park—wherever we are alone with our thoughts.

As we tell our story to ourselves, we select out those pivotal events, no matter how insignificant they may appear to be, and those symbols of our past that will help us to steer a course into the future. When we do this, the past and the present coexist side by side in our mind. We carry with us an awareness of how our past life influences the moment in time we are in now. It is because of memory that our life has continuity. We filter these memories, and from them we create our own continuity.

Penny, in coming to terms with over ten years of infertility, reconstructed her life story around a sense of difference from others. She described herself in childhood as being like everyone else, living a typical existence in a small rural town. But starting when she was 16, the events in her life made her feel different from others. First, her father died suddenly. Her mother, incapacitated by grief, was unable to care for her children. So Penny took on the job of looking after herself and her two younger sisters. Her father's death drastically altered the family's economic situation and put an end to her plans to go away to college.

Then, when she was 19, she began having severe pain near one ovary. Barely able to function, she finally went to a hospital emergency room, where she was told she had a cyst on her ovary, and was diagnosed as having endometriosis. The physician she saw told her that pregnancy sometimes stops the progress of the disease, and recommended she not wait too long to get married and have children.

This dramatic incident, following closely on the heels of her father's death, had a profound influence on her life plans. She had been planning to marry her childhood sweetheart someday, who was in college several thousand miles away, and someday after that to have children. Suddenly, she was filled with a sense of time galloping past her and having to reorganize the whole plan for her life. So, instead of marrying someday, she and George married when she was 20. Both families were upset. George's family withdrew their financial support. She moved 3,000 miles to be with him and worked to support them while he finished school. Instead of waiting until her late twenties to conceive, as she had planned, they started trying when she was 21. When she was 24 and he was in graduate school, she became pregnant. She went back to work as soon as the baby was born. Because the threat of endometriosis still hung over them, they began trying to conceive a second child one year later, in spite of their financial difficulties. Penny finally conceived for the second time when she was 33.

Penny felt forced to reorder her values because of her endometriosis. She had been raised to see the person she thought she would become as a different person—as a woman with a college education and a career *before* she married and started having children. Having to rewrite her whole life script at 16, followed by fifteen years of being focused on her fertility, affected the way she viewed her whole life.

> We have never fit in. Infertility has made us different all along. Because we knew having children would be difficult, we got married and started trying when everyone else was single. None of our friends when George was in college were planning to settle down anytime soon. They thought we were strange. We didn't fit in then.
>
> And now, the people my husband works with have a single lifestyle, so we don't fit in with them, either. Our values are different from theirs—we are family-oriented. And our families want us to make them grandparents, and point out how all our brothers and sisters now have big families. They just don't understand infertility. They have never "gotten" it. So that makes us different. It has always been like this—we don't fit in anywhere. We never have.
>
> We have finally given up trying to fit in. And stopped apologizing and explaining why we have a child who is so old, when we just now have a second one on the way. We live our lives to suit ourselves, and we don't have too much contact with our families. So that helps.

In reworking her identity, Penny has moved beyond the sense of stigma she initially felt when she was diagnosed with endometriosis, a feeling that has recurred over the years when she has felt glaring differences between her lifestyle and that of others. She has woven her sense of difference into her identity as a strength, a testimony to her unswerving determination to live out the high value she has always placed on children and family. In constructing and reconstructing her life story, which has changed over time, she has managed to maintain her sense of self-consistency in the face of significant life obstacles to her goals.

The life structure Penny anticipated at 16 was torn down around her through the death of her father and the diagnosis of endometriosis. At 33, through her conscious development of her own life story and the positive interpretations she has put on it, she has developed a new structure for her life. This new structure emphasizes the values that are *really* important to her, values she is passing on to her oldest child.

> I worry I have warped our daughter's values. She thinks having children is the most important thing in the world. Sometimes I feel guilty that I have given her this message so forcefully, but at the same time, that's what I believe myself. So I feel like I am giving her my values. I want her to have these values. They are important to me.

One of the tasks of mid-life is the restructuring of our values. In the beginning of this book, I talked about how values are reshaped at mid-life to better express what men and women want from life. This process of rethinking values doesn't wait upon a diagnosis of infertility or some other life crisis. It proceeds, with growing momentum, as we pass through our thirties and into our forties. When a woman or man faces a major life problem, it precipitates a serious review of values, no matter at what age the problem occurs. If the crux of the dilemma appears to lie with an inability to live up to the old values, it is necessary to give our values closer scrutiny and refine them so that they better serve our needs.

> The unexamined life is kind of tragic to me at this point, having examined mine in such minute detail. I had a real review of values about my family. I dug them up, I examined them, I rejected some, and I kept others. I feel like I'm a different person. It was like going to a shopping mart, a shopping center of emotions and prejudices and values and deciding to discard some and retain some.
>
> —Greg

In examining ourselves so closely, we begin the individuation process, the gradual realization of the self over a lifetime, in which we increasingly strive to find out who we *really* are and what we *really* want from life. This process never ends. It goes on for the rest of our life.

Not only does the struggle for individuation go on ceaselessly as we move through life, the way that we address problems in our life and the efforts we make to resolve them may change for good. As we age, we turn increasingly from problem-solving through action to problem-solving through a more internal process of reflection. Part of this process has to do with what we learn as we mature—that sometimes there are no answers that are exactly right, and that many of the decisions to be made in life are really compromises.

This is certainly true of infertility, which reinforces the need to turn to inner resources to successfully cope. More and more we come to realize that how we view an issue has to do mostly with what is going on inside of us, with our identity, with our values. We learn it's a matter of perspective.

> I should have never let that happen to me—that feeling that I had lost my identity. The group leader kept talking about reclaiming the self. And I have been working on that. But maybe that happens to women in general, even women who have children and stay at home, and you lose your self, and then your kids leave home.
>
> I think you have to feel viable. If you break things down in percentages, I don't want my strongest identity to come from my aerobics class or something like that. I don't value that. But I can't say I visualize myself as four kids and a full-time mom, and real into it that way, either.
>
> I feel the old person is coming back. It has been a good summer. I think I will look for my career to help me cope. At work I am asking them for change. And find fulfillment in doing other things. Like my pottery. I love sitting at the wheel, watching my hands shape the clay. And feeling the answers are coming.
>
> —Theresa

IDENTIFYING LIFE THEMES

Anthropologist Sharon Kaufman has observed that people usually develop themes that capture the essence of their lives. These themes can be anything. There are themes of hardship and themes of hope, themes of discovery and themes of steadfastness. Women and men usually have more than one major theme running through their lives. These themes may represent two or more different sides of themselves. For example, when things are not going well, a person may live out the theme of "not good enough," and when everything falls into place and goes well, the same person may live out the theme of being "special."

Jeff had several themes in his life. He contrasted his slow, steady approach to things unfavorably with his wife's ability to go from one idea to the next, from one career to the next, with flair and creativity. He saw himself as the boring partner in this relationship.

> I'm a plodder. I'll kind of go after something and slowly build on it. I do things in a straight line, whereas Sarah—she has this ability to grasp an idea and take it in all sorts of directions, then let go of it and go on to the next thing.

But being a "plodder" was only one theme. Another theme that he described in talking about himself was "pushing the limits."

> I like to push the limits of everything, just to see how far it will go. To see just how far you can push something until it breaks. And then you know, okay, in the future you can only go this far. But until it breaks, you don't know how far you can take a concept. You have to test it. And I like to test things.

In the process of rethinking his identity and developing his life story to fit with the next stage in his life, Jeff came up with a third theme. He saw this theme as "overdoing it."

> I'm the kind of person who goes in one direction too much. If I make a bowl of chili, I overdo the hot sauce. I overdo everything I do. I don't know if it's to make a point, or why I do it.

Searching for his own inner balance between these various themes, Jeff decided, after putting much energy into his infertility and its treatment, that he wanted a child by any means, that donor insemination or adoption would be okay. He thought a child would balance his own life, and give him perspective. And he saw the road to generativity as being lived out through a child.

> I kind of decided that the best thing in my life would be to simmer down, change my focus. There are a lot of things I could do to do that. I think having a child would be a great way to pass on some of the things I have learned, and a lot of the mistakes I have made. And simmer me down some in the process. Kind of help me refocus my life and get off my own kick so much. It's kind of funny, because when we started with this whole thing, I didn't care if we had a child or not.

Like Jeff, we have the power to transform the themes in our lives. If you are asking yourself, "What are *my* themes?" start thinking about your own life story. What are its themes? If you are feeling depressed, chances are you will become gloomier as you remember the important losses of your life and attach negative meanings to them, as Marsha did when she said, "Everything I touch turns to poop." This is a theme. Many people, especially when they are dealing with feelings of failure about their fertility, express these kinds of sentiments.

If you have asked yourself a lot of soul-searching questions, and you think this, or something like it, might be one of your themes, then it's time to review your life story again. This is something you may be doing on a daily basis, anyway, if you are in the midst of a search for the meaning of your life. Embellish your story, fill it out, put in whatever is important to you, no matter how small—*all* the people, *all* the action. Look for the positive, the hopeful, even while you are facing the difficult, the impossible.

Ask yourself about the pivotal events. *Why* were they pivotal events? These events could *appear* to be insignificant, for example, the day you climbed the flowering apple tree and sat amongst its blooms, the night your parents started fighting during dinner and you had some revelations about your family. You probably have a host of memories of all different sorts, with different kinds of feelings attached to them. Ask yourself, what were *all* your feelings about them, not just the dominant feeling, whatever it was. That dominant feeling is important, and it may be the one you remember first. You may carry it around with you. It may even be at the crux of your major life theme. But it may also camouflage other feelings. And, just as important, it may hinder you from taking a more objective look at your subsequent experience of life. It may be self-defeating, and hide your sense of mastery from your own view.

A lifetime of negative messages from her family led Laura to accept a theme her family had chosen for her—the bitter spinster. So enveloped was she in this theme that she could not see any of her positive qualities.

> My mother made it very clear to me at a very early age that I was just like my aunt and would undoubtedly grow up to be like her—this angry, bitter, manipulative spinster. So I knew I would never get married, never have children because she didn't. I couldn't allow myself to think about it. My mother and my aunt did a real number on me—I was absolutely, totally convinced they were right.
>
> But I wanted to lead a happy life even though I was always alone. I went into therapy with only one question on my mind, 'Can you get me to break out of my belief that I am going to grow up to be just like my aunt?'
>
> When I got married, at the age of 35—about as late as you can get—that was one of the greatest days of my life. Imagine, somebody I cared for wanted to marry *me*!

> But the fertility problem is like a replay of all my mother's messages. So it's back to square one. Then you tell me this is useful, talking with me about infertility. It made me feel wonderful, and part of me said to myself, 'Intellectual, verbal woman that you are, of course you are good at this crap. You talk everybody blue in the face about anything that matters to you.' If I can do something about this issue, if I'm articulate enough that I can make some changes, that really makes me feel good. It gives a purpose to my life.

Like Laura, you can find a positive theme within yourself, one that describes you. Often, this theme is the descriptor others use about you as well—the way the world sees you. It may be hard to connect with these positive descriptors of the self if you have a fertility problem. Fertility, when it is not actualized through an easy conception, has a way of canceling out all the good feelings we have about ourselves.

What are some positive themes you might find in yourself? Not surprisingly, the first themes we think of usually reflect our cultural values. They arise out of the spirit of rugged individualism and fierce independence from which our country grew. When it comes down to it, it doesn't really matter from which ethnic or religious group we spring. Because sooner or later some of these values are internalized by all of us, in one way or another.

Here is a list, a handful of adjectives and phrases. Do any of them describe you at any time, either now or in the past? Do any of them reflect the way you see yourself now or have ever seen yourself, even for some brief five-minute period?

Indomitable	Self-sufficient
Resilient	Autonomous
Independent	A seeker
Determined	Individualist
Self-reliant	Special
Able	Unique
Competent	Likable

Down-to-earth
Fair
Diligent
Loyal
A survivor

Everyone should be able to find some part of himself on this list. If you can't find yourself there, you have temporarily lost the most important part of you. Talk to your partner, or to a friend, a relative, or a professional. Work at finding this missing piece. Because everyone has a side of herself that conveys something positive, no matter what. If you are having a hard time seeing the valued side of yourself, it's time to turn to others for help.

You may have other words you like better. These are just a handful of the positive attributes Americans believe in and use to describe themselves. If you have other words or phrases that carry more meaning for you, what are they? Fill them in, instead. The important thing is to find out what your life themes are. This list is just to get you going, to start you thinking along these lines. Your list, when you are finished, may look very different from this one. That is good, as long as it reflects you. It is just as valid.

This is an exercise in self-discovery, in developing your life story. I believe that our life story, whatever it is, can give us insights into how to handle our transitions in life. Your life story can provide you with insights about why fertility has become such an important topic in mid-life. It can give you guidelines for how to cope with the issues you face. And it can be a reminder of your strengths when you are feeling ineffective.

But everyone has a different story, so I can't write you a specific prescription for how to do it. A professional, seen face-to-face over time, can help you find your own guidelines and get this process under way. The only alternative is to think and feel it through for yourself. I can only give you the tools, and a little push in the right direction.

If you think this approach sounds Pollyannalike—if you have been delving into your darker side in seeking the light—that is probably where you need to start. When we can look at the dark side of our lives—at the not-so-great things, the losses, and the pain—it's because we *need* to do it. When we confront the worst things that have happened to us, or the worst things we can see in ourselves, and we come back to them time and again, there is a reason. That reason lies within the self. Usually it's something we have to work our way through before we can see light at the end of the tunnel. Whatever the trigger—whether it's the equation of bleakness in our lives now with some episode in childhood, or a job that's hard to face each day—it's not going to dissipate until we take a closer look at why we feel this way.

When men and women seek their life story by looking at their dark side first, they can benefit from professional help, simply because looking at this side of ourselves can lead to depression and despair, if there isn't someone guiding us toward the light. We may get stuck in the same ruts we have found ourselves in before. Or we may become preoccupied with the sheer awfulness of some of our life experiences. We may, as a result, cast negative aspersions upon ourselves. We may tell ourselves that the worry about being a terrible person underneath it all has come true.

As I discussed at the outset of this book, when we initiate plans to parent, we do so because we want to re-create the family. But starting one's own family is an invitation to the ghosts from the past to enter our inner house. And when it doesn't work out the way it was planned, our ghosts get agitated, and they stir up all kinds of things, mostly forgotten, that have retreated into the corners of our mind. They go through our internal house like a whirlwind, toppling over our dearest memories and tampering with our equilibrium. So when infertility strikes, it's necessary to lay these ghosts to rest, however we can. Otherwise, they will stay to haunt us.

If you come from a family that wasn't "typical" in some way, a family that had its problems—however you define them—then you may benefit from some other voice who can help you to address your family issues. If you're not comfortable with a therapist or counselor, consider listening to the voices in the books currently available to adults trying to understand the riddle of their family life. These books may help you to find your own answers, so that you can rewrite your life story.

You may have a negative life theme that often seems like it is running your life. And you may have a positive life theme that is being played in a much more minor key. But sometimes you can't hear that music at all, not even faintly, because it has been drowned out by a negative theme that seems to be engulfing you. This experience is common to women and men coping with fertility issues. It often has to do with relationships between the generations, both now and in the past, with family rules and ways of being that have been handed down to us by the generations that preceded us. Our family plays a big role in the formation of our life themes, as Laura found to her chagrin. But it is not necessarily the case that you must take drastic measures, as Jeff did when he left home, in order to find your positive themes and leave your ghosts behind.

Composers have taken this idea of themes to heart in writing operas. As the curtain rises, the "light theme" is dominant. But as the play proceeds, when plans go awry, the tragic tones of the dark theme grow in intensity and gradually take over, erasing the light theme altogether and preparing the audience for the tragic end.

Don't let your story turn into the makings for an operatic tragedy.

In order to transform your life story and transcend this crisis of mid-life, you need to reverse the order of these themes, so that positive themes are in the ascendant. If you work at it, you will eventually be able to turn this phenomenon around, so that you can live out your positive life themes, with only a minimum of interference from your darker side. Marilyn, whose story I told at the beginning of this chapter, did this. So did Carrie, and Penny, and Jeff.

You can do it, too.

CHAPTER 13

REMAKING ROLES

It used to be that couples became parents early in adulthood. By the time they were in their early forties, children were spreading their wings and preparing to take off, leaving the door open and the family home echoing in silence. This phenomenon led social scientists to coin the term "empty nest" to describe the phase of life women and men entered in their forties, the time by which childbearing and rearing was expected to be over.

It's a little daunting to those of us who don't fit this mold to open a book about mid-life and find that the only kind of issue being considered is what to do when the kids leave home. What if we haven't had children yet, or think maybe we won't after all? What yardstick do we measure our issues by? Women and men feel at odds with their own culture when they are out of step with the timing of life stages. But it's not the person who is out of synchrony—it's a statement about how fast our culture is changing. Without an accurate crystal ball to gaze into, social theory usually plods tardily behind the changing culture.

The empty nest is a swiftly fading phenomenon, as ever greater numbers of women and men rethink their roles in life—their potential as parents and ongoing changes in their careers. When the empty-nest syndrome was given its name, women's work was in the home, and men's immersion in a career was expected to be total. The "empty" part supposedly belonged mostly to the woman. Even though the marital relationship was affected by this transition, a woman's loss of direction was viewed as the problem.

Women, whose career was once seen as in the home, have moved into the marketplace. At mid-life a woman is likely to have rewarding work outside the home regardless of whether she has children or not. Most women with small children do work. The stay-at-home mom is a person from the past—from our parents' generation—unless she is a New Age stay-at-home, who decides to retire at 40 after a lengthy career.

Marsha had been working in a high-level administrative job that she disliked for years. She was good at her work, and it paid well. But after a number of years she basically saw her work as a way of biding time until she became pregnant, at which point she planned to retire from the field she was in. Then it was discovered in a routine medical procedure that Marsha, a DES daughter, had a small uterus that might affect her ability to conceive and carry a pregnancy. She was plunged into rethinking her career.

> When you have a deformed uterus, you think, 'Oh, my God, I'm going to be working in this place the rest of my life.' I really want to get out of there. But if I'm not going to be a mother, then I have to work.

When fertility is questioned, women and men take a closer look at their roles—the ones they live out routinely as well as the ones they have been unable to fulfill easily. This unexpected life transition is a challenge to roles, a challenge that coincides with mid-life concerns about how to live out the balance of one's life.

Each person goes through life with an agenda of where she wants to be in mid-life, a mental list that constitutes self-actualization. At this stage of life, it's not just women who may want to retire, or look for change. Men, too, reconsider their goals and their interests. They change careers, they return to school.

Larry, in an effort to come to terms with the crisis he and Susan faced, began rethinking his roles.

> You're supposed to have a job, whether it's being a garbageman or a steel-welder or a teacher or whatever. You're supposed to be married and support your family. And do all

> these things. And if you don't, you're very deviant. Sometimes I feel trapped by that, trapped by my own ethic, that I was brought up with and bought into.

The ferment caused by fertility issues leads women and men to question themselves, and where they are going in life. As they approach the critical midway point in their journey, they realize that half of life has passed. They ask themselves, "Have I reached my destination?"

The idea of what is self-actualizing changes as we go through life. Not only do women and men differ in the amount of gratification they experience in different roles, their expectations about those roles change as they live them out, for example, when a woman who once enjoyed her career and planned to remain childless changes her mind and decides to pursue pregnancy.

Theresa, rethinking her direction in life, weighed her current job against her long-term plans.

> For the last four years I think, career-wise, I have not really challenged myself. Especially since I didn't have a family. If you have a family, you get fulfillment out of that and feel like you don't need a career. But I feel like I don't have either.
>
> I don't know what's going to happen in the next couple of months. If adoption works out and we decide to go for that, then what I'm doing is fine. I can work with the baby in my arms. But if absolutely not—if there were not to be a child in this house—then I definitely would need to find something more challenging. And really commit myself to something I could do.

Women's and men's mid-life markers of what constitutes satisfying roles may not completely mesh. It's not that couples don't share goals. But even when they do, priorities are different at mid-life, when they are concerned with getting it right—getting their lives together once and for all.

One-sided cultural expectations for women and men create

conflicts that have their roots in the culture itself, since cultural norms have historically dictated that women nurture, while men achieve. Women, as carriers of responsibility for the family life cycle, have internalized this conflict between nurturance and achievement. When fertility plans do not proceed according to schedule, women come face to face with this dilemma, as Paula did:

> There was a time in my fortieth year after my birthday when I was just depressed all the time, and a lot of it centered around the fact not just that I was 40—if I'd been 40 and pregnant it would have been okay—but 40 and a body that doesn't work just threw me much more than I ever anticipated. I hated my job. I wanted to get pregnant so I could have a year's maternity leave because I wanted to get the hell out of there.

Women are forced to address the meaning of nurturance for themselves and their roles in mid-life. If they are not going to become a parent and nurture children, what will they do? All women facing infertility ask themselves this question.

INTEGRATION OF THE SELF

Jung was the first of many theorists about the course of life to suggest that at mid-life women first discover and explore their instrumental, force-in-the-world side, while men become more expressive and begin to get better in touch with this side of themselves. This theory has been borne out in cross-cultural studies of men and women in mid-life. The effort to bring the different poles of oneself into closer proximity to create a more balanced self is a process that begins in mid-life and continues for the rest of the life cycle.

Fertility issues dramatically introduce these tasks of mid-life.

When men and women dig deep into the self to meet their own and their partner's needs, they stumble over previously overlooked parts of their life work. For men, the task often begins the process of excavation of the self and integration of it with the more developed, instrumental side. For women, the task may be to integrate the expressive and instrumental parts of the self into a cohesive whole. Carol Gilligan has suggested that integration of the self takes place in a different way for women than for men. Nevertheless, the task for each is essentially the same, turned inside out.

Theresa ruminated about her lack of direction as she sought her self:

> I think it was a mistake, not pursuing my career. But I don't have the motivation to just go out and find a full-time job because I don't want to enter into something and be overcommitted to it.
>
> The career is an area to work on to get my identity back. I know I can do it. But I don't put a high value on it right now. I think the whole superwoman thing is a big mistake. You can point them out in a crowd. I think it's a killer.
>
> If I could resolve the infertility one way or the other, I think I would be more likely to throw myself into deciding what to do. I can't remember feeling this stuck for a long time. I know I have a lot of energy. People describe me as hyper, and I know it. I can still talk a mile a minute. It has not destroyed my personality, but my energy to accomplish anything is gone.

Because of the recent tendency for women to delay childbearing and seek achievement in the world, the work of integrating the different parts of the self may have already begun. But only begun. What is missing becomes apparent when a woman's attempts to conceive are not initially successful. She must continue to work on the integration of these different aspects of herself, a dilemma that all women in our society face at some point in mid-life. The timely appearance of children may simply postpone the task.

Paula described what happened to her:

> My best friend and I were at work, and we were working on a schedule for me, and I burst into tears. I said, 'I can't do that—I can't be here that much. I don't want to see this place.' And she was just shocked. It was like falling into a deep hole that I eventually started crawling out of on my own, without getting pregnant.
>
> When I started putting the pieces back together again, I realized I was okay, and that if I couldn't get pregnant, that was okay. What was happening was I was becoming increasingly okay. I feel differently about my job now. I made some changes to it, and now I'm happy with it. I have no desire to leave.

This is one of the final tugs of war in the battle of the self that women experiencing infertility face. Virtually every woman I talked with had experienced a crisis around her career and the meaning of her life in dealing with her fertility. This was true for women with highly successful careers as well as for women who bemoaned their lifelong lack of career focus. The bigger issue for each of them was creating a successful merger of the two sides of themselves, a merger that has been consistently discouraged by cultural attitudes about what women's "true" work is.

As time passed, Theresa felt increasingly ready to turn her energy away from her infertility and get on with her life. Six months after she reported feeling stuck and unmotivated, she began making major changes in her life.

> I'm feeling good about the direction I'm going in now—the way I'm starting to feel more involved with my work whether or not I get pregnant. That feels real good. I'm asking them for change. So that whole thing is growing. I'm even starting to think about working full time.

As women begin to find themselves, they may be gripped by enthusiasm, even excitement, as new possibilities in life open up. As she began coming to terms with her infertility, Carrie began to see her life differently than she had in the past:

> I'm trying to further my career. It's exciting. A child will complicate all that. Of course, I would juggle both of them. I wouldn't give up my work if a child came along. But I'm not going to say that a child is the only focus of my life. I have other things in life to look forward to.

A woman's career does not usually become a major issue in the relationship, unless she doesn't verbalize it and her partner observes her turmoil and imagines it to be related primarily to him. It is therefore important for a woman to articulate her career issues. This is one area in which her partner can really provide support and is unlikely to feel seriously threatened. Theresa was reassured by Paul's support:

> We talk about it. Paul says, 'You shouldn't put your life on hold; you can't let having a child dominate your life, you can't let it steer your life.' And I can agree with that. I think he's right—it was a mistake to get sidetracked professionally.

Because men compartmentalize careers away from family issues, verbalizing these concerns will not threaten him. He will probably see them as separate from himself. Not only that, he has gone through life having career concerns of his own. If there is any issue he can relate to, this is it. He can offer his partner not only sympathy but useful ideas for how to approach the issue, as well. Talking to Russ about her career helped Carrie to develop a new perspective:

> I began to look at my career in a different light. Russ has been really good about that. He's had to deal with it himself.

Not only that, his struggles with his own career may mirror hers or interact in a way that may strengthen the feeling, "We're in this together." If he is going through a career crisis, she is in a better position to offer support herself, provided, of course, that she can put her own preoccupations aside to listen to his problems.

Men who have a crisis in their career, especially if it coincides with the discovery of their own infertility, undergo an inner crisis that may seriously affect their identity and serve as a catalyst for mid-life issues of the self to emerge. Celia described what happened when her husband learned he had a low sperm count:

> Ron and I made an appointment with the head of urology, and he said, 'Look, these results aren't good. If I were you, I would think about alternatives.' Five days later, Ron lost his job, so he kind of hit bottom.

This crisis forced Ron to take action to deal with the situation:

> Then, during the time he was unemployed, he went to the bookstore and got a book on infertility. He started to think about things more. It was Ron who called Resolve to ask about groups.

Celia, reflecting on how this crisis ultimately affected both Ron and her, said:

> It was a terrible blow. I think that, compounded by losing his job—I don't know—the two things together seemed to really open him up. It was at that point that we stopped fighting and got on the same track.

When men are simultaneously hit by infertility and by problems in their career, achievement in *any* direction seems stymied. This *is* the crisis of their life, and support from their partner is essential to weather this assault on their manhood. When a man's partner is able to offer support for his dilemma, it becomes a building block for the relationship. When partners meet each other on these issues, they strengthen the bond between them, as Jenny and Matt did:

> MATT: I waffled on whether to change jobs. And finally I did change jobs. But I was so preoccupied with our infertility at that point that I made a significant mistake and almost got fired.
>
> JENNY: And me, if I hadn't been so emotionally strung out over the infertility, I would have been able to handle the politics of my job. Instead, I put my foot in my mouth, and didn't get promoted. And then I went on to a job that was a pressure cooker.
>
> It was a time of tremendous upheaval. But in the process, something happened in the dynamic between us. Because I don't want to blame our infertility on him. It's very complicated, but I think we have grown together.

CHAPTER 14

THE QUEST FOR RESOLUTION

> I've been pushed to my emotional limits. Being infertile is like being the walking wounded. I refuse to minimize it, anymore. I'm going to do whatever I need to heal. Hopefully, I can make some good come out of this. I need to feel hopeful.
>
> —Holly

Hope is what propels us through life, no matter what our life situation, no matter what we hope for. Our culture is oriented to the future. When we can no longer foresee a future for ourselves and feel unable to proceed to the next phase of life, we become emotionally trapped in the present. Life feels as if it has come to a standstill. That sense of motion through time has stopped. Its loss throws our equilibrium out of kilter.

Infertility symbolizes the loss of the future. It is not possible to move on with life until the future has been reorganized in a person's mind and given new meaning. On the broadest level, resolution necessitates finding what was lost: the meaning in life. The life story must be constructed to fit a different set of circumstances than those originally anticipated. To do this entails the preparation of a place in the life story for an altered set of hopes and dreams.

In this reorganization process, new room is created—freed up for new and different kinds of hopes and ideas to be entertained. If the new possibilities are found acceptable, they are incorporated into identity.

The process by which hope is transformed and men and women move toward resolution is a gradual one. It happens little by little. Sometimes the day-to-day process may seem very ordinary. Susan and Larry reflected on what it is like:

> SUSAN: I feel like resolution has been happening, even though I guess in some ways we have less of a decision now than we did six months ago when we were going to stop treatment at a certain date. It's resolving itself. It's not a resolution. It's ongoing. It's not, Did it happen? No, it's something that just goes along. It's working itself out okay.

> LARRY: That's the best we can say for it, I think. It's sort of squirming along. I think maybe it's a lifelong process. Every day you go forward, and you put these different experiences under your belt. You get a little greater perspective. It's like biorhythms. You're not sure where it all swings on a given day.
>
> I think there's a progression. We are further along the continuum than we were before, although even that's not absolute—it doesn't exclude outrageous behavior! Maybe that's the best way to put it.

Susan and Larry are clearly on the road to resolution—together. What goes into resolution? Resolution is made up of many ingredients. One set of ingredients is comprised of all the contents of a person's life that have been sifted through, sorted out, and viewed in a new light. A second set of ingredients are feelings that have to be acknowledged and consciously experienced in order to be digested. A third set of ingredients involves the relationship, and the work that goes on between partners as they move toward unity. The sum of these changes in each partner and in the relationship equals preparation for resolution.

Resolution itself seems to occur in a series of interactive stages. Most women and men go through several specific phases as resolution draws close. The first of these is a complex process in itself: letting go of old hopes.

LETTING GO

Letting go of hope really starts when a person is able to acknowledge a loss and begin mourning it. It is not just the loss of the perfect child, it is the loss of not getting life on terms of one's own. Mourning the loss may therefore start fairly soon after things begin to go awry. As time passes, precisely what is mourned changes. As the process of accepting loss ebbs and flows, women and men adjust their perspectives to this shift in their field of vision, as Dierdre did:

> I don't think I'll ever get over being infertile, but maybe sort of living with it, like an old friend. 'Well, here it is again—it will pass.' You know, things like that. Just learning to tolerate this incredible pain and becoming a little more balanced. Sort of tempering your excitement and also ignoring your depression a little bit. That helps.

Letting go is a process that may take years. It usually has many subtle stages as well as some definite turning points that are unique to the individual. Each person has a unique life history. This history is a significant part of the resolution process, since reworking this experience into a life story that makes sense of the inexplicable takes time. Sandra, recounting how this process occurred for her, traced how different events, big and small, contributed to her realignment of hope.

> I started talking to other women about their symptoms, and it's clear that we had similar symptoms—that I am premenopausal. That brought up the aging process. And I thought, 'Oh, my God, this is my change coming—very quickly.'
>
> When I was talking to these women in my group, they said, 'Everybody's different—what did your mother go

> through? What was her menopause like?' And I remembered her hot flashes very well because they were very intense and it all happened very fast, and she went on estrogen. My mother was always very young looking—people were always commenting. Then the aging process started, and she aged very quickly. It happened when I moved away from home. I went back a year or two later, and she had stopped the estrogen, and I remember being so shocked at how my mother had changed. When I remembered all this, I really began to think about my own aging.

Then, in the midst of dealing with the fact that she herself was aging, Sandra got a phone call saying she should come home. All her issues escalated:

> My sister called to tell me I'd better come home to visit as soon as I could because she didn't think my mother would be around much longer. And at the same time she told me she was pregnant. My mother has been in a home, and we suspect she has Alzheimer's disease. My fantasy over the past two years has been finally getting pregnant and going home and telling my mother the news. And when my sister told me, that was another step in having to accept it. I had to go see my mom and let go of that.
>
> It took me a month to resolve that and be able to go home and just let that be. That was a big step in the whole process of letting go. I have felt an enormous release of energy since I came back.

But that wasn't all—there was more. Having been forced to face some difficult realizations, she was primed for further insight into herself. Soon after she came back from her trip, she had an enlightening conversation with a friend.

> A friend has been talking to me about her miscarriage and how she felt it was her fault. And it brought up all kinds of

> feelings about my own miscarriage ten years ago and the enormous guilt I had been carrying around about it.
>
> My friend said, 'The doctor was assuring me that it was my body's own way of letting go of a fetus that probably wasn't right to begin with.' I felt such relief when she said that. I remember so well the relief that I felt when a doctor said that about my miscarriage, and I reexperienced that relief.

Sandra was puzzled by her own response to this conversation. Why did she feel relief, and what did it mean for her life now?

> I asked myself, 'What was that all about—that relief?' And I realized that I could apply it to myself right now. That that was another step to forgive myself, that somehow when it comes down to it that I am responsible in some way. And feeling guilty about it. And also feeling that maybe I am deeply ambivalent about having a child at my age, but I have not been conscious of it. I have such a conscious yearning and such a sadness around not having one that it's really hard for me to believe that I could be saying no.

The jolt of learning about and acknowledging her own mixed feelings gave her another way of looking at her relationship with Tony and her part in the complexities that had developed between them.

> I think the way I kept it unclear with Tony, and kind of let it go, was part of my deep ambivalence. Out of fear. I was not using every opportunity I had to get pregnant. Enough has gone on in my life that would create these feelings of fear.
>
> So I started thinking about it in a whole new way. And that was when I was able to start grieving and get myself ready to move on.
>
> And having to come to terms with myself on the deepest

> level and saying to myself, 'It's for the best—it's for the best. Okay.' And I *can* be a full, productive person.

Not everyone is forced to let go of cherished dreams in the dramatic way that Sandra was. Letting go is often experienced as a much more gradual series of subtle transition points, as Larry and Susan described. Regardless of how women and men let go, once they do, ways open up to redirect and transform hope.

Sandra was suddenly freed to alter the course of her life. What did she want to do? She decided she wanted to adopt.

> It certainly feels to me more settled and more clear than it has before, that I want to put my energy into adopting and I couldn't do that until I reached a certain point in feeling that I wasn't going to have a child of my own.

On another level, letting go involves rethinking one's basic philosophy of life. The death of loved ones at this time of life invariably brings this issue to a head, as women and men come face to face with issues of their own mortality. This is another step in the process of integration and an important part of the resolution process, as women and men give up impossible hopes and put fertility issues into a broader perspective.

Laurel, as she worked at resolving her miscarriage, reexamined her philosophy of life in the context of her entire existence. Questions about the meaning of life rose to the surface as she explored this no-man's-land of difficult issues and emotions.

> You wonder how many losses you can take. For most of my life I didn't have any tragedies and I didn't really experience a loss, so you think that everything is okay. You think life is all right, and then, all of a sudden, you pass that threshold and you are on the other side, and you realize it isn't wonderful. I still haven't resolved that.
>
> It's hard dealing with loss, and I think I'm just going to

> have to get to the point where I accept it. It's something that people just don't talk about, so you are kind of alone.

This is one of the main issues of mid-life, recognizing and coming to terms with our own ultimate mortality. Because people don't talk about issues like these, we may feel alone. But experiencing the solitary nature of the self is part of the process of the mid-life coming of age. Laurel's review of her life involved coming to grips with life itself. Looking into her own depths from the solitude of the self enabled her to identify what was meaningful in her life, and reaffirmed the importance of connecting with the people she loved.

> My way of resolving this has been to take a cosmic point of view. Hopefully, life will become more meaningful because you know there is an end—you just can't postpone things. So I have been trying to make more of an effort to not let things hang and to let people know that I do love them. That's hard. I wouldn't say I've gotten too far but I think I've taken the first step in just being aware of it. Trying to resolve conflicts as I go along.

Part of letting go lies in rethinking what generativity means. Generativity is what we make of it. We re-create ourselves by passing to others our storehouse of knowledge, our beliefs, and our values. Our ability to share our life experiences with younger generations gives meaning to our life. Is it necessary to have children to do this? There are many other ways to be nurturant, to experience the fullness of life. Reflection on this issue often starts with thinking about the next generation, as it did for Susan:

> We went back to my hometown to visit my family, and it was the town's bicentennial celebration. There was a pancake breakfast on Main Street, and all their neighbors and friends were coming up to us, and then there was a parade. It was all about the history of our town. I was on the edge of

> tears the whole time. And I wondered, 'What is this about? Why am I feeling so teary and sad?' Finally it hit me. History of our town. Generations. Children. None.

Even as she was resolving her infertility, this experience led Susan to struggle anew with the question of whether or not a life without children would mean an incomplete life cycle. As she sorted this issue out, she recognized how much of it remained tied to cultural expectations about childbearing and childrearing.

> I keep running up against these assumptions from people: 'You'll never be mature unless you have children.' It's not something you argue with people about because it's sort of emotional—a moralistic value of our society.

She saw that resolution, for her, meant overcoming this prejudice—a prejudice that she shared with others.

> I really had to wrestle with that. A lot of the earlier psychologists back that idea up, you know, Freud especially. It isn't until recently that there is much support for how you really can grow up and be a mature human being without having children.

The recognition that she was challenging cultural assumptions about what people do in life prefigured her resolution of the problem. It enabled her to differentiate between her own wants and the need to fit in and be socially acceptable to others.

> That's a big hurdle. When you start challenging all those assumptions, all of a sudden you start to look at the interplay of yourself with others, like, 'How much of it is whether I really want kids or do I want to be like my other friends who are having kids?' Then I ask myself, 'How much am I missing nurturing and raising an individual child? And how much of it is missing all the attention I would get for doing that because it is socially accepted?'

After contending with this problem over time, the wishes of others, once identified, became less important, and the need to please herself, first and foremost, grew. When Susan sorted these issues out, an underlying concern was revealed: her ambivalence about having children.

> Sometimes I feel like, 'Yeah, I really do want kids,' but I know the other side is there, too—the ambivalence.

Once the ambivalence that was originally experienced at the beginning is rediscovered—before the decision to have children was made—it frees women and men to let go of the old hopes and to ask themselves, "What do I want *now*?"

As Susan mulled over what generativity meant to her, time passed. She gradually moved away from an intellectual, objective perspective to the question, what was the meaning for her own life?

> I ask myself, 'What does it do to this sense of progressions and the sense of continuity with the generations, and the feeling that you are leaving something beyond you?' I'm trying to bring it down from being an ideal that I'm losing to just being a different reality.

Letting go of ideals and accepting a different reality is what resolution is about. Once the clutter of old hopes—including the hopes and expectations of others—has been swept away, a pathway is cleared on which to proceed into the future. As she prepared to make this transition, Susan concluded,

> I think probably my parents' generation will never deal with it in a positive light, but I think *we* need to—we need to find positive ways to incorporate infertility into what we think about adult life.

REINTEGRATION

Once they are able to let go of their old hopes and dreams, men and women are ready to move on to the next step. They begin the process of integrating this experience with the rest of their life. Integration means reclaiming the self and putting together all the changes—in the self, in life expectations, and in daily life. Once they are integrated, they become part of a new foundation on which to build one's life.

As women and men begin to reintegrate their new selves with the old, they must ask themselves the same questions again: "What do I really want? What are my needs? What is the next step I need to take for myself?" This is a giant step. Except that it doesn't usually feel as big as it is. Because with this step comes new hope.

> Things are different for me now. Here I am, at a point where the grasshopper has to become an ant and start making preparations for the future.
>
> —Al

An important part of the resolution process is the integration of the old self with the new aspects of the self—the parts of a person that have changed in undergoing this crisis in mid-life. We don't necessarily become different people, but we may look at life and at ourselves differently.

As Greg looked back, he saw how many changes he had gone through and how he continued to experience the differences in himself on a daily basis—changes that affected the whole fabric of his life.

> For a while I took the attitude of, 'I need to have an answer. Either I'm a father or a kingpin.' If I'm going to be a father, then I don't want to be building up a big business that is

> depending on me. I don't want to be building up an economic network—getting on and off planes, building an empire and doing things that will be both consuming and satisfying, a place to keep my hands busy while I wait for infinity to take over.
>
> Then, after a while, I started asking myself, 'Wait a minute—what are all these agenda items? What are all these expectations that I've got to do this or that? Why can't I just say, Maybe I'll try a little of this and a little of that?'
>
> This is sort of what I'm going through now. I don't have to do adoption, but it's something I can look into. I don't have to do much more medical treatment unless Gina absolutely insists. I don't have to work. It doesn't have to be 'something.' It doesn't have to be an either/or—an extreme.

What were the consequences of these revelations? Greg's new approach meant he had to reevaluate his entire life in relation to himself.

> Infertility has forced me to confront my value system—of everything I've thought about, believed in, my prejudices—everything. It has made me reevaluate every aspect of my life. Business is business. It's not loaded with this other agenda. I'm a more quiet, self-assured businessman now. I do things a little less stridently. I'm proud of doing a good job. I will not compromise my peace of mind or the peace of mind of my staff. I am there to enjoy it, not to shove it down their throats.
>
> I don't volunteer. But now I have. Types of friends, economic status, social status, sexual orientation—and all the other things—they have all been sort of reevaluated. I think infertility was the catalyst for me getting to that spot.

Generativity and the New Self

Part of teasing out the new self lies in rethinking how generativity applies to one's own life. When Greg described his new perspective about work, that was about generativity—what he could contribute through his work—doing a good job, enjoying himself and his fellow coworkers.

What needs to be resolved at this stage of life is, on one level, the place of children in a person's life scheme. Women and men learn through their experiences that generativity is much, much more than a child. Nevertheless, this question must be addressed by both men and women since parenthood is viewed as bringing completion to this stage of life.

> I had really finally gotten to the point where I accepted—*mostly* accepted—what was happening and it would be all right not to have another child. I could live with that and be okay. I felt like I was getting more on an even keel, so to speak.
>
> —George

Susan's resolution of her infertility made it clear that nurturing children was important. Having reached this ultimate realization, she and Larry began to consider adoption.

> I'm coming to a time where it seems more and more clear we are not going to have our own children. From a rational point of view I can see there are a lot of other things you can do that will accomplish exactly the same goals, but emotionally it is still hard for me to accept for myself that that would be as good. And feeling I would be missing out on some developmental phase.
>
> It's like an emotional thing that is hard for me to let go of—it is hard for me to accept for myself that childlessness would be as good, that it would be okay. It's the idea of what I am supposed to do as an adult.

By this time men and women have evolved a more individualistic set of values that enables self-acceptance to occur. They have modified cultural values to be congruent with their own life experience. This is essentially a process of "destigmatization," in which they reject the sense of stigma they formerly associated with their infertility. Stigma is no longer relevant for where they are going in life.

Ultimately, the process of integration leads to reconnecting not only with the self but with life. It enables men and women to move beyond the roadblocks to intimacy and friendship that are created by fertility problems and the other issues of mid-life.

> After we adopted and it was on TV, a friend taped the show and brought it to the annual golf tournament. A lot of old, hard-core guys, thirty or forty of them, were watching this tape, this seven-minute tape, and we were all in tears at the end of the tape. A bunch of old rowdy guys.
>
> The tape addressed the issue of infertility. Nobody made any rude comments or anything like that. So I guess we talked about it in that fashion.
>
> —Kenny

CHAPTER 15

REACHING RESOLUTION

Resolution is a gradual process that occurs on many levels over a period of years. In a sense, all of life is an ongoing quest for resolution, as we strive to resolve the issues at each stage of life in our passage to the next set of life tasks.

There is no formula for how long it takes to reach resolution. Everyone is different. Not only that, each individual goes through the different phases that lead up to resolution at a different pace. The longer it takes to recognize a sense of loss and begin mourning the loss, the longer the entire process will take. If medical treatment has been undertaken, the nature and length of treatment affect whether, and how, loss is perceived.

Other life events intervene in this process, as well. These events may help in the final process of resolution, as they did for Sandra, in confronting her own and her mother's aging process. Or they may be a distraction from the work of resolution, and retard the process.

Women and men often worry because they feel unresolved and long for resolution to occur so they can go on with their life. They are tired of their inner struggle. Sometimes it seems endless. When a person feels this way, he is usually in the midst of the resolution process already, doing the work necessary for resolution to occur. Grieving, exploring other options, constructing the life story, finding new outlets for self-expression and creativity—all go on in the midst of the inner dialogue that retools identity.

RESOLUTION AS A COUPLE

Couples often reach resolution at about the same time. The amount of change they are processing simultaneously may feel exhausting, as Jenny and Matt found out:

> JENNY: It turns out we're just not going to have children in our relationship, and that has been something that has taken seven or eight years now to roll around to. It's just what turns out to be.

> MATT: That's what happened. I think Jenny and I would be good parents. But this is what we've got, and this is how it is.

> JENNY: At a certain point I just had to decide that this has taken up too much of my life. I'm going to go on with life. I can't devote any more special time to the situation. We just don't want to do it anymore. We don't want any more strings. It's too exhausting.
>
> It was such an upheaval. The whole time was. We don't want any more of that. Now we sort of want to sit around and be peaceful, and have friends over for dinner, and walk on the beach. It feels like we have to heal up from what was a tremendously emotional time.

Jenny and Matt were experiencing reintegration as individuals at the same time that their relationship was taking off in new directions. The possibilities seemed limitless.

> MATT: I'm changing careers. I've got applications in all over the country. I'm thinking over all the possibilities.

> JENNY: It took a long time to get past the fertility stuff, but

> that's just how it goes. I figure I gave it my best shot, and that's all I can do. It really interrupted my career. So I'm getting on with my life. I have other things to do.
>
> I ask myself which direction I should take? I look out there at the sky, and there's a lot of space. That's sort of how I feel. Like I'm surrounded by all this empty space. I love having all this space. It's an incredible feeling. I feel like my life's ahead of me. I can fill up as much of the space as I want, or not. It's up to me.

In their struggle with infertility, Jenny and Matt have discovered something critical about themselves: They have learned that the meaning of life lies within the self. It is up to us to create our own meaning—to discover that *we* have meaning in and of ourselves. No one else can do it for us. Only we can unlock it, only we can recognize it. But once we have, we can enjoy it to the full. We can embellish it, deepen it, and watch it grow.

This is the mid-life search for the self.

Resolution is not a straight path. It may feel like a forced march over windy and crooked roads, through dark forests and deep rivers, across dry stretches and over high mountain peaks. But eventually, the burden you carry will lighten and the answer will come.

> It was wonderful to see in the Resolve group, couple by couple, people coming to a resolution, and what a difference it made. Even if the resolution was not what they had hoped for, it mattered. You could see people become transformed just by deciding not to pursue something anymore. That was really something to watch.
>
> —Celia

What the answer will be for you depends on you and your partner. No one else can predict what it will be. In the pages ahead I give examples of different kinds of answers—answers that worked for people in this book. Perhaps they will help you to find your own answer.

ADOPTION

The big issue for most couples who face infertility is whether to adopt. Men are usually ready to contemplate adoption before women are. Adoption means a woman loses the experience of pregnancy and childbirth. And in addition, it removes her sense of bodily control over the process. Adoption becomes the Great Unknown, and women, especially, may be very fearful of it. Most women must resolve these issues before they are freed to seriously consider adoption.

Couples may remain out of step for a long time because women approach this alternative slowly, while men, who see a plausible solution, often become impatient. They want to get on with their lives. Adoption usually becomes more attractive to women if time passes and the likelihood of a biological child diminishes.

Adoption itself is not hurdle-free. Both partners must contend with the lack of control they may feel over the process, and with the shortage of available children. The prospect of the significant efforts they must make to acquire a child, whether through agency-sponsored or private adoption, may be daunting.

Dorene did see adoption as the ultimate alternative, but she expected to get pregnant. She never thought she would reach the point of actually adopting. She and Kenny began to seriously consider adoption when their medical options dwindled. They made an appointment and visited an attorney who handled private adoption.

> It was a real interesting experience going to that interview. I remember feeling that I didn't think it was going to happen. I had gone through so many disappointments that by this time, even though I thought I was going to get pregnant, I also didn't think I would be so lucky to do it. So I thought after all the infertility, adoption would never happen, either.

They started the private adoption process, which begins with sending out letters to various parts of the country in search of a child. Four days later, they got their first response, which didn't work out, and then a few days after that, an aunt in another state called to say she knew someone.

> We ended up contacting them. They were teenagers. They wanted to give the baby up. Private adoption wasn't legal in their state, so she decided she wanted to come live with us for the last few months and have her baby here. We decided fine. Before that, whenever we talked about it, we had decided there was no way we could even meet a birth mother—that it would be too traumatic. But as time went on we got more and more desperate and accepting of the process. We thought we had to jump at anything that came along. We got more phone calls after that, but we had made a commitment.
>
> So she came to live with us. And that was real stressful. She was very homesick, very young. She was breaking up with her boyfriend. It was mass hysteria. She wasn't eating the right kind of food. It drove me crazy. It was a wild experience. I don't know if we would do it again—we do have this gorgeous little girl here. But it was really hard.

It got harder when the birth mother changed her mind.

> We were right outside the door when she was born, and we heard her say, 'Give her to Dorene.' There was no hesitation. From the outset she said, 'I don't want to see the baby. As soon as it is born, I want her taken out of the room.'
>
> Two days later she went back home, and *then* she decided she didn't want to give her up. But she didn't do anything about it. She kept putting off signing the relinquishment papers. That went on for six months. I was just terrified they were going to come get her. Finally, she signed.

Dorene and Kenny wanted more than one child. They decided to adopt again in about three years. When their daughter was about eighteen months old, they got a call from their original letter. This adoption experience was very different.

> When we got the call, I said, 'We are interested in adopting again, but we have this baby,' and the social worker said, 'Oh, that's great because the birth mother wants her child placed with someone who has an adopted child.' So she put us in touch with the birth mother. She had already picked out a couple, but it wasn't working out. She had decided to interview some more couples. She decided we were the ones.
>
> She was absolutely wonderful. An entirely different experience. We felt really good about her. She had gone through counseling. It was a beautiful experience with her. She said when the baby was born she would want a few days with her. But the day she was born, she said, the heck with waiting. Come down and see her, so we did. And the birth father was there, and his mother. It was a little bit crazy. The grandmother was crying. She didn't want them to give her up. But they did. They are still together.
>
> It was a neat experience. We all sat around naming her together. And when we left, the birth father came up to Kenny and was saying, 'You are going to be the father of my child.' It was just such energy—real positive.
>
> And off they went. We heard from them a couple of times after that for business kinds of reasons, like 'I want you to know I signed the papers yesterday.' No fooling around. We did that adoption ourselves, without a lawyer. Now both of them are final.

Now that both adoptions are final, how do they view it?

> Before we adopted, I wanted for us to have a child of our own together, even if we adopted. Now I feel these two are the children of our spiritual making, the children of our

> heart. I believe we produced these children through our love rather than through sex. So to me it's the same thing—they are children produced from us.

LIFE WITHOUT CHILDREN

Another option, although a more difficult one for many women to contemplate, is going through life without children of one's own. Remaining childless, however, is a viable option for most—though not all—men. Somehow, remaining childless may seem like a very different way of going through life than what women and men have been contemplating for their future, although that is the way they have been living their lives until now.

Theresa was seriously considering being childless. She had given it a lot of thought, and spent much time talking to Paul about it.

> The leader in Resolve really wanted to talk about child free. She wanted everyone to say one positive thing—just try it on—what would be good about it? One woman really couldn't do it.
>
> Maybe I'm someone that needs to not put all my eggs in one basket as a way of salvation or protecting myself, saying, 'Well, this is a possibility.' So I had some experience toying with that idea. I have a husband who thinks like that, too. You have time to do other things, travel. My sister will tell me a million things—why I wouldn't want it.
>
> That doesn't mean I'm unloving, I think. That was something that came out in the group. Like maybe you don't really want kids, you're not really maternal. But it doesn't mean that, I don't think. It's just another part of me.

Theresa came from a big family, and had a lot of children in her life already. She planned to build on these already-existing relationships with her nieces and nephews.

> I'm loaded with nieces and nephews, and I find that really helpful. My sister is real concerned about me in kind of a neat way. She is a good support. She is worried about me in a real loving way. And her kids are great. For some people I hear them talking nieces and nephews . . . it makes them sad. But for me, I really love my nieces and nephews. I could be this great aunt.

Theresa envisioned other kinds of generativity that went beyond her involvement with other children and her interests.

> Another reason I'm open to being childless: I don't think about it in terms of who is going to be there when I'm old. I assume, watching my grandmother and Paul's grandfather, I will get involved with other people and be a doer, and just be active.

DONOR INSEMINATION

When a man has an infertility factor but his partner appears to have no fertility problems herself, donor insemination (DI) becomes another option. Most often, it is men who balk at this possibility—the idea of another man's sperm being used to create a pregnancy. Most, though not all, women find DI an acceptable alternative. If men are able to get past the idea that DI is an insult to their masculinity, this option may contribute to a highly satisfactory resolution of the problem for both partners.

Celia and Ron joined Resolve after a crisis when Ron lost his job and learned about his low sperm count almost simultaneously. They began to explore different options.

> After I'd been in Resolve a while, adoption seemed like an alternative. It was a different point of view, like we *could*

> have a baby instead of maybe we will. I don't think I pushed for donor insemination. I wasn't sure how I felt about it, either. I told Ron I would like to be pregnant, but I didn't really push it at all. I backed off.
>
> I don't know how he came around to it, but one day he said to me, 'I'd like for you to have a baby. I'd like for you to be pregnant. It's okay with me.' So we contacted the doctor who does artificial insemination and we had to wait to see him. They wanted us to bring pictures.
>
> So we brought a picture of a camel and a rhinoceros, and we gave those to him. We all sat there and laughed together. It was pretty easy after that. It only took three inseminations.

When couples choose DI, women worry that their partner will feel distant from the child, and that this distance will impede total acceptance of a child as a man's own. Celia was no exception.

> I worried because I was on bedrest before the baby was born. I had nothing else to do. But he has always seemed to love him. He has seemed very much his baby from the first. He always held him more and was very watchful. Yesterday he said, 'Who could deprive anybody of having Jimmy as a sibling?' So I think he is wild about him.
>
> People have said that Jimmy looks like him. I think those are the most awkward times, but actually, I think he does look like him. If he had any trouble getting attached to him, I think it is gone.

What does having a baby by DI mean for the future of their family?

> A few days ago Ron said, 'Now the only thing to consider is if we will have a donor next time, or if there is anything that can be done about me.' In a way that makes me a little

> nervous because I am worried that he would love a baby who is biologically his more than Jimmy, but in my heart of hearts I don't think so.
>
> So I'd love it if I could have Ron's baby, but as far as I know, I can't—we can't. It doesn't mean we can't have a wonderful baby, and a wonderful family. And we do.

ADVANCED REPRODUCTIVE TECHNOLOGIES

Most people start considering advanced reproductive technologies only when they have exhausted other, less expensive medical treatments. Eileen and Roy had been married for ten years and trying to conceive for five years before they seriously considered trying in vitro fertilization (IVF).* About the same time, they began looking into adoption. Eileen said,

> We started going to Resolve's adoption seminars, thinking that the IVF percentages were low, anyway. But because our insurance paid part of the IVF, we decided to try that. Otherwise, we didn't think we could afford to do both. What if the IVF failed and we had spent all our money? We thought we would do one, and see how it went. The decision to do IVF was mine, because he really didn't care. He could have done adoption first. He said, 'It's you taking the drugs. You decide.'

Roy interjected, 'Well, she was going to go through most of the grief, so I left it up to her."

*In vitro fertilization (IVF) is an advanced multi-step procedure in which multiple eggs are stimulated by the use of combinations of fertility drugs, removed from the ovaries transvaginally by an ultrasound-guided needle, then mixed outside the woman's body with her partner's sperm. The fertilized eggs are

Eileen said,

> So we did three IVFs, and then we got really serious about adoption and started working on our letter. But meanwhile, we were sort of a textbook case. Every time they would say, 'You're having absolutely the right reaction, you're producing this many eggs, you fertilized this many, and this is like a textbook.' We didn't have any other odd medical problems to cloud the issue.
>
> But it didn't work.
>
> I couldn't decide if I wanted to do the fourth IVF. I was very ambivalent about the whole thing. I just kept thinking, 'I can stop anytime. I'm really not commited to this until the actual transfer.' So we composed our letters. Did the pictures. Ran around having people take pictures of us. Went to an adoption symposium. We sent out our letters, talked to an attorney, then we started with an adoption agency. Then I did the IVF. And once I did it, I said, 'I'm glad I did it.' Because now it's out of my system. I don't want to do it, anymore. I don't care anymore, it's not that important.
>
> When I was having second thoughts about doing another IVF, I started to think, 'This is just too much of a hassle. I need something that will produce a baby at the end, and adoption will.' It helped that neither of us was dead set on a biological child. We had had a plan in mind if that IVF didn't work, how we'd proceed with adoption. So we did that, and now we're taking infant care classes, even though we don't have a child in the picture yet.

Similarly, after a great many other medical procedures, Cyra and Geoff decided to try advanced reproductive technologies.

---

allowed to incubate and if developing normally, are then transferred transvaginally into the uterus for implantation and an ongoing pregnancy (Robert D. Nachtigall and Elizabeth Mehren, *Overcoming Infertility* (New York: Doubleday, 1991).

Their physician suggested gamete intrafallopian transfer, or GIFT,* as it is commonly known. They had one adopted child but they wanted more children, and Cyra wanted to experience pregnancy. She said,

> I went through a lot of things. I had years of taking my temperature. I did maybe a year of clomiphene, I had a laparoscopy. I had unexplained infertility. Then we decided to do GIFT. They extracted a bunch of eggs and they just fertilized some of them, froze the others, put these little guys together in a dish, and plugged them back in. But meanwhile, we started to think about adoption. We were moving towards GIFT and adoption almost simultaneously, but we were still hoping that GIFT would work. It was a lot of energy and a lot of money, and we felt we weren't getting anywhere. I didn't know I would go through with it until the day that they did the egg retrieval. I really wasn't sure. I was very ambivalent about it. I wasn't ready for another disappointment. And I was very frightened of the procedure. I had had somewhat of a traumatic experience with treatment a year before that. I was really sure it wouldn't work. But the insurance covered it, and that pushed us over the edge. So we did it. They extracted the eggs. They got a lot of eggs, they fertilized the eggs.
>
> But it didn't work the first time. So we did it again.

Geoff interjected, "Everything was working out very well the second time. I was optimistic. I had no pessimistic feelings at all. I mean, I didn't necessarily feel it was going to work, but everything was going according to plan."

*Gamete intrafallopian transfer (GIFT) is an advanced infertility treatment that involves the placement of a mixture of eggs (oocytes) and sperm directly into the fallopian tubes. The procedure involves a number of steps, including medications to induce many eggs to develop, the preparation of sperm, the retrieval of eggs and the placement of a mixture of eggs and sperm into the fallopian tubes, usually through a laparoscope (a microsurgical tool) (Nachtigall and Mehren, *Overcoming Infertility*).

Cyra said, "I was doing it to get control over my life. I didn't believe it was going to work. And then it turned out I was pregnant with triplets, and I lost one. One dissolved or was absorbed. One didn't make it. So we have twins!"

Reflecting back on this experience, Geoff said,

> When you go through this process, where you go through adoption first, you realize that it doesn't matter whether this child is linked to you biologically, because in all other respects it's your child. Then when you have your own children biologically, you realize, who knows, they could be serial killers, or God knows what. You don't really have that much control. It just blurs that distinction entirely.

DONOR EGG

I interviewed Clara and Connor after they conceived by going through a donor egg program, using an egg donated by another woman.* They had been going through infertility treatment for a number of years. Clara recounted how things had started:

> Fifteen years ago I got pregnant through an IUD when I was 21, and I had an abortion. So I thought I could always get pregnant. Then five years ago I developed pelvic inflammatory disease, and I had a right ovarian abscess and they took the ovary out and the tube out and the left tube was com-

*Egg (Oocyte) Donation allows women whose ovaries are unable to produce fertile eggs to become pregnant. This includes women born without ovaries; women whose ovaries have been damaged or removed because of endometriosis, infection, or tumors; women whose eggs did not fertilize after undergoing in vitro fertilization (IVF); and women whose age precludes treatment with their own oocytes. A young egg donor is given injections of a combination of fertility drugs to increase the number of available oocytes, these oocytes are removed by transvaginal needle aspiration, and the oocytes are fertilized with the sperm of the recipient's partner. The fertilized eggs are then transferred transvaginally into the uterus of the recipient for implantation and an ongoing pregnancy.

> pletely blocked. And there was a lot of scar tissue. So that was that. That started our fertility quest.
>
> Over the next few years I had several surgeries, and we did three IVFs. They failed. Meanwhile, we heard about donor egg at a symposium, and we asked our doctor about it but he wasn't set up to do it so he referred us.

Asked what their initial response was to using a donor, Connor responded,

> It was a poor second choice, in my opinion. We were going through second choices and lining things up, and they became increasingly disagreeable. I really wanted to just remain a family. If it wasn't going to be Clara's, at least I wanted it to be her sister's egg so it would still be family. That was a major concern. That was our first choice.

Clara said,

> But she didn't want to do it. She's very young, and she had never even had a pelvic exam. So she backed out. And I was starting to become resigned to doing donor egg. It became obvious it wasn't going to work with my egg, and so what we saw as possibilities were child-free, adoption, and donor egg. Actually, that was exciting for me because the success rate was a little higher than regular IVF.
>
> So we went for an interview with this specialist and did a donor cycle and it failed. It was tough. We were devastated, and we didn't come up for months. Finally, I had more surgery. I had been putting it off, thinking I could get around it. But in order for me to do this fibroid surgery, we made a deal, the two of us. We had to do at least two more fresh cycles with a donor and we had to start working on adoption. We had to start working on a letter because I didn't want to get to the end of our fresh cycles, frozen, or whatever they were, and have to start from scratch.

> Then we tried to use our frozen embryos and they didn't survive, which was difficult. Because most donor embryos are reused. That really threw us because it was like coming to the end. It's hard to keep going.
>
> So finally we called our donor and asked her if she would do one more cycle with us. She had experienced a lot of pain with the last retrieval. So she agreed. And we went through with it.
>
> And . . . I'm pregnant, 24 days.

Overwhelmed by her emotions, Clara burst into tears. Connor took up the story: "We're really excited. Apprehensive. We've hit the wall before, and it took me months to recover from the last one. But I'm fairly optimistic. Yeah, real up. I announced it to my entire class [of fellow graduate students]."

Recovering, Clara said,

> We haven't been very private about this whole thing. We've been very open about using a donor. We want to educate people and we're not ashamed of it. This is an option for a lot of people. It's not cheap, and it's pretty emotionally wrenching, but it's another alternative. And until recently it didn't exist. So we like the educational part. We volunteered to talk to people through Resolve, and we get calls from all over the country. But the main thing is I really want it to work.

I went back to visit them when the baby was almost due and asked Clara how she felt about having the baby now. She responded, "I knew I was pregnant but it took me a long time to believe I was going to have a baby. It was probably not until like the seventh month. I mean, long after the baby started to move. Now that the baby's almost here, I can finally get excited." Turning to Connor, I asked how he felt about becoming a father in a few weeks. He responded, "Its a mixture primarily of extreme excitement and total terror. It's something we haven't done before."

THE UNKNOWN FUTURE

Sometimes things happen when we least expect them. Susan and Larry put a lot of work into resolution. They looked at their alternatives. One was remaining childless. Susan thought this might work out for her, but it was Larry who was most enthusiastic about the possibilities.

> We've thought about it a lot. So far it has been pretty good as a life, so not having children is sort of a continuation of that. We've talked about getting pilots' licenses, and getting a little airplane and start traveling around and doing things. There's a lot of things you can do and have freedom. It's not looking at life as being childless, but being very full in other respects.

They also considered adoption, about which they had been thinking off and on for several years.

> SUSAN: We talked about adoption for a long time. We could have done it when we were working overseas. But we weren't ready. And lately, I have been feeling ready, but then I hang back.

> LARRY: But now that I'm looking at jobs in different parts of the country, we think we will wait until we move and are settled down again.

Meanwhile, Susan decided to go to graduate school and finish her training as a psychologist.

> I applied to all these different schools. We don't know where we will end up, but we decided it wouldn't be a good idea to adopt while I'm in my first year of graduate school. So we'll wait and see. We stopped feeling the time pressure we used to feel. Who knows what we will want to do in a couple of years?

Susan was accepted to the graduate school of her choice, and Larry was offered a challenging job nearby. They moved, and launched into their new life. To her complete surprise, Susan learned she was pregnant in her second year of school. Their daughter was born into a family life that had been regeared for adult living. By that time, Susan was immersed in her graduate studies, and Larry was deeply involved with his work. Neither was willing to give up the newfound interests to focus solely on parenting, as they had been in the past. What did they do?

> We manage to fit everything in, but sometimes it's a struggle. It's been a challenge. Life is so unpredictable. You just never know what lies ahead.

CHAPTER 16

WHAT LIES AHEAD

> When you see people who have not gone through this process as far as you have, you begin to recognize that it *is* a process. At first you just think it is misery, you don't know it is a process and that it seems to have steps and that there is growth and acceptance—that something is going on here. But when you start talking to people who are at different stages, you begin to see that. It helps.
>
> —Gina

This passage in time is part of the journey through life. But its path is so thorny, it's hard to see that we *are* traveling, moving from one stage of life to another. The journey is made more arduous because it seems the future is just beyond our grasp. In order to reach it we must come to terms with so many inconsistencies—both within ourselves and in the outer world. Yet one by one these inconsistencies become resolved, as we rework our life script and rebuild the structure of our lives.

If you still feel swamped by the loss of the future, it is no consolation to be reminded that time will pass and you will be swept into the future, like it or not. Time really does march on, a truth that persons facing fertility problems are painfully aware of. It's moving into the unknown, impersonal future without having secured the personal future we have planned that's hard to bear. It seems at times that we are drifting into a directionless, purposeless void.

This is why you may feel trapped in the present and why it's important to mobilize your energy to get past these shoals, on which you may feel that you will be eternally grounded. They *are* a trap, but one of our own making.

When we take the reins and find our direction for the next stage in our life, our sense of mastery over our own universe is restored. Our feelings of competence are renewed. And, most of all, we start feeling in charge of our own life again.

The first task is to find your direction as an individual. But following hard on the heels of that task and, indeed, interactive with it is finding your way as a couple. The goal, as a couple, is to come out of this leg of your life journey within arm's reach of each other. The *fear* is of coming out of it poles apart.

But the fear is seldom realized. When partners seek themselves and pursue their needs as individuals and, at the same time, communicate with each other about their feelings and concerns, they move in tandem toward the goal.

In this book I have tried not only to take you through the odyssey that couples undergo in search of fertility, but to provide you with benchmarks along the way, ones you can cling to, if need be, when the undertow threatens to loosen you from your moorings. Ulysses's odyssey is, in a very real sense, analogous to what the journey through infertility is like. For there *are* sirens out there, in the form of stereotypes men and women hold about each other, that threaten to blow us off course. And there are becalmed waters—times when it seems impossible either to move forward or to turn back.

Throughout the book I have tried to give you guidelines to move you safely past these and some of the other dangers that lurk in the shadows. Some of these suggestions are aimed at you, the individual, while others are intended for your relationship.

Here is a brief recap of the main points. Some of them may look different—perhaps more feasible to explore now—than they did at first glance.

ACKNOWLEDGING THE DIFFERENCES BETWEEN YOU

You could sit down together and just talk—about what you, as a man and a woman, want from life. This is a conversation without end. You can renew it daily, weekly, monthly—whatever feels right.

You can explore, together, all kinds of things—what it's like to be a woman, what it's like to be a man. You can examine how your own gender may affect your thoughts and feelings.

You can tell each other how you feel about the expectations and pressures you feel you are under—from each other and from the society in which we live. You can talk about the past—growing up and adulthood—and start to weave together a new sense of your continuity as a couple. And you can talk about your vision of life and whether or not it has changed.

You can also talk about your fears—in general as well as those specific to your current situation.

All these things, and more, you can, and should, talk about.

There's only one thing you should try *not* to do. It's both big and important to work very hard at each time you talk—and all the rest of the time as well. *Try not to blame each other.* Remember, this whole situation is nobody's fault.

Avoiding blame is a good general rule of thumb to follow, anyway, but here I am talking specifically about blame based on gender, such as, "He doesn't understand—he's a man." This sort of thinking will get you nowhere. Like the rational/emotional stereotype, it's another way of discounting your partner and making things worse. And as someone who has experienced infertility, you know what it's like to feel discounted. Don't fall into this trap.

OTHER KINDS OF COMMUNICATION

There are all kinds of ways of communicating with each other. Sitting down and talking is only one. It's very important. But what happens when one of you wants to talk and the other one doesn't? During times like that, consider using the 20-minute rule, in which the person who wants to talk can do so for 20 minutes and no more, unless the partner wants to continue the discussion. This is a helpful way to allow one partner to say what's on his mind, without his mate feeling overburdened by another, possibly endless, discussion.

What about fighting? Couples fight. It's a fact of life. A relationship without arguments—that's free of fights—is not necessarily a healthy relationship.

There are many ways of expressing disagreement, verbal and nonverbal, through thought and action. Indeed, disagreement with each other is healthy and is human. We are individuals, first and foremost. It's critical to express feelings. For many couples, fighting and arguing are the only way to get in touch with how they feel and to learn what their partner is experiencing. They may shout at each other, or cold-shoulder each other in icy silence before they finally start to talk. Or they may cover the whole spectrum.

What about angry feelings that are unexpressed, that sit and smolder? Some couples may not really know how to fight. They may discuss issues very politely, yet feel hurt or angry inside.

Whatever your own pattern is, you have probably learned how to handle anger and disagreements more effectively as time has passed. The question is, Are you effective enough? Do things get resolved? Do hurt feelings linger? Does each of you feel attacked? Are some of your exchanges irretrievable, threatening the relationship with permanent damage? It is important to evaluate how you are both handling your anger and pain, and to seek help, if necessary. A professional can help you sort out your issues and teach you to communicate with each other more effectively.

My other advice relates directly to infertility:

1. Don't use infertility as a weapon. Infertility is no one's fault, so there's no point in blaming the partner; for example, "If it weren't for you, I could have a child." Try not to indulge in self-blame, either. It's equally fruitless, such as, "If it weren't for me, *you* could have a child."

   If you have the urge to use infertility as a weapon, ask yourself, "Why?"

   Equally destructive is the Unequal Eagerness Bind: "He doesn't care if we have a child or not." Don't get caught in this. It *is* a bind. More is happening here than just imbalance in the desire for a child. Lines are being drawn between you, and stereotypes are being set up. It's another form of blaming, of finding a target for anger that doesn't go away. The problem is, not only does the anger not go away when this happens, it grows, becoming a cancer that can infiltrate the entire relationship. It can polarize partners along gender lines, trigger dysfunctional coping patterns, and in general, wreak havoc in a couple's life together.

2. Don't fight in bed. Or near the bed. By this I mean don't involve sex in your fights at all. It doesn't matter how physically distant you are from home at the time. You may be sitting in a doctor's office together, or get into a fight in the parking lot. If the topic of the fight is sex, it doesn't matter where you are—you are treading thin ice.

The tragedy that may befall a couple's sex life when anger is injected into a situation that is no one's fault was outlined in Chapter 5. It has many forms. Work as hard as you can to not poison sex with anger. It's a hard job because sex may be very stressful right now, along with the rest of life.

Monitor yourself and your feelings. Explore how you feel in your depths. Talk with your innermost self. Then put yourself in your partner's shoes. Remember, men and women may view sex differently from each other when they struggle with fertility. But regardless of these differences, sex has enormous symbolic meaning for both of you. Its importance in your relationship should be acknowledged, time and time again, if necessary. Talk with your partner *before* sex gets loaded. And having started, keep on talking. Don't wait until it's too late.

GETTING BEYOND STIGMA

Stigma is part of culture. All over the world—in many different cultures—people experience stigma in response to some cultural expectation—some way in which they feel they don't measure up. Infertility is universally stigmatized, so there are people who feel as you do in every society about their inability to carry out their part in perpetuating the species. If you feel this way, it may help to know you are not alone.

But stigma is more than a fact of life. It is a virus that pervades culture. It's unhealthy, but it's hard for people who have some negative characteristic assigned to them to avoid. Stigma promotes bad feelings about the self. It feeds inertia, it fuels anger and resentment. It has the potential to poison our belief in ourselves.

In order to move on with your life, you need to disown the stigma you may feel. This is a necessary part of the process of integrating the new self with the old. As the new self—the changed you—emerges from its chrysalis, it is essential to leave behind those aspects of the former self that endanger the healthy self being reborn. Feeling stigmatized is one of the main things you must try to leave behind.

A sense of stigma necessitates redefining what is normal. In order to get beyond stigma—to free yourself from its constraining yoke—you must take yourself through a process of "destigmatization." Essentially, this involves separating the stigma of infertility from you, the individual. How can you do this?

You can start by revoking certain cultural attitudes, such as the belief that people who don't have children are "not as good as" those who do. Beliefs are not truths. Cultural beliefs are sometimes neither healthy *nor* accurate. They *do* represent the norm—those things that characterize the majority of people's experience. Being outside this norm is what makes people feel different from others. It's what makes them ask, "Am I normal?" If you have felt the burden of being outside this norm, it's time to start looking at yourself and the situation differently. Remember, being outside the norm and being "normal"—whatever that is—are not the same thing.

A Step-Wise Approach to Overcoming Stigma

First, examine your own values. Maybe they need to be retuned, as I suggested in Chapter 6, to fit the reality of your life better. Maybe you have been buying into societal values too much in an effort to conform, and not allowing yourself to develop a more individualistic set of values. There *is* variation in cultural values. Not everyone is stamped from the same mold to share identical values. It would be very boring if we were. Ask yourself what you think, what you value, as a result of this experience.

As our identity changes, so do our values. This process is somewhat like the adjustments we make to the camera lens when we take a picture. This is part of our adaptive capacity as humans, to alter our behavior and our ideas to fit our changed life circumstances.

Once you have begun the process of realignment of your values, you will feel greater self-acceptance. You can then proceed to handle other people more effectively.

Second, it's up to you to make the rules. There are no rules for etiquette about infertility. Create your own.

If you are miserable because of what others are saying or what *you think* they are thinking, remember that they act out of ignorance. Don't become a martyr. You have a choice: You can educate them, or you can ignore what they say in the knowledge that you know best. In other words, you can discount the importance of their attitudes, as you may have felt discounted by them. Don't be a slave to cultural attitudes.

As I said at the outset of this book, culture is a strong force in our lives. It *shapes* our lives. But every individual must work out for her- or himself a path that balances cultural expectations with self-acceptance. To do so restores our faith in ourselves, our sense of who we are. It reaffirms our identity.

Third, remember that you are not alone. Millions of people in the United States are in your shoes. People who face the same problems and have the same sorts of experiences as you do with fertility issues.

As hard as infertility may be for you to talk about, talking to others who share your experience is crucial. It helps to talk with others about something we have in common, especially something that troubles us. When we face stigma in our lives, it is critical to connect with others who share our experience. Talking with others defuses the stigma. We find out we are not alone. We begin to see ourselves differently, no longer as lesser than others. For most people, this is the beginning of letting go of stigma.

Get involved with a self-help organization, such as Resolve. It may help you begin to see the whole problem of infertility differently. If this option is not available to you, or if the idea of joining a group of people is difficult to consider, start by seeking out another person you know or suspect may share your problem. Or you can call a Resolve hot line—for people in crisis—and talk with someone anonymously. Or ask the professionals you know working in the field of infertility for other suggestions and resources.

If there is no one you feel you can talk to—if you feel truly alone—seek the help of a counselor or therapist. Remember, privacy and secrecy are two different things. Infertility is too big a burden to carry alone.

It may not be possible, or even desirable, to put the experience of stigma behind you completely. Once we have experienced stigma, it becomes an indelible part of our identity. But you can incorporate it into your identity so that it becomes a positive force—a sort of repository of knowledge—in which you store the idea of what it is like to feel different. This is knowledge you can put to use throughout your life—without having it poison your ability to be effective. In time, you may come to see your experience of stigma as a strength that helps you to face other life experiences.

MAKING LIFE NORMAL AGAIN

Although infertility may initially appear to be a minor inconvenience in daily life, it grows in intensity as our emotional investment in finding a solution grows. As time passes, we may find ourselves in emotional limbo that seems without end.

Have you postponed big and little changes in your life, changes that could make a real difference to your sense of well-being? Many people do. They put off moving, whether it is across the street or across the country. They hesitate about job changes. They procrastinate even more about career changes. They even put off vacations because it may mean the loss of a reproductive cycle. Believe me, this is no time to put off a vacation with each other!

If you have been procrastinating about making decisions in your life, ask yourself, "How long has this been going on?" If you have been putting off major decisions for over a year, it may be a major contributor to your feeling stuck.

Then ask yourself another question: "How much does my lack of movement affect my everyday mood?" For example, if you are bored to tears in your current job but it would be perfect if you had a child, ask yourself *again* if it is worth it. It's probably *not* worth it and may be contributing to the problem. When children come along, women and men adapt to cope with the demands on their life *then*.

Live your daily life in the present, not the future. Change what needs to be changed. Not living life to its fullest now because next year things will be different just isn't good enough. Life is for living every day. Don't fall into the trap Lisa fell into: "I have been infertile for ten years and have nothing to show for it." Don't give up a year of your life—or even six months—if you can help it. What if you look back in ten years' time and ask yourself, "What did I do with my life when we were trying to conceive?" Don't let the answer be "Nothing."

How to Make Life Normal Again

If one or both of you are suffering from inertia and can't get moving, work together on how you can start moving along in life again. Start small, by getting away on weekends together, by taking a vacation.

When you are alone together and away from the daily grind, review your life plans—*all* of them—not just the plan to become parents. This was never your *only* goal in life, was it? Most people do *something* in life besides have kids. And those who focus solely on parenting later complain that life has passed them by. Having children *isn't* everything, although it does seem that way right now. Try to remember what your other plans were and start putting them in motion.

Another way to break out of inertia is to seek out new interests. Explore your creativity. Ask yourself what you enjoy doing or would enjoy doing—it can be anything. Did you do it in the past? If you did but you stopped, ask yourself, "Why?" Maybe now is the time to get back into it.

If you think of something that interests you but it's totally new, try it out in a supportive, nonthreatening environment. Evening classes in a community college are a good place to find out about new interests, and they keep you from sitting at home, depressed.

Another way to break the cycle of boredom and depression is through exercise. As long as they like the type of exercise they are doing, exercise makes people feel good about themselves. It makes them strong and healthy. It fights depression. In a few years' time, if you're chasing after a toddler, you're going to need all the strength you can muster. So you could look at it as a reserve bank account for the future.

As you start to make life normal again, ask yourselves as a couple, "What do we enjoy doing together?" If you haven't spent much leisure time together lately, what did you once do that you enjoyed? And start doing it. Chances are, preoccupation with fertility has put a cramp in the pleasure you used to get from each other's company. Infertility has a way of doing this. Boredom can be poison to a relationship, just as virulent as anger and resentment.

If you and your partner have been suspended in time, start today to break out of your time warp and get on with your lives. The richness you create in your life now will benefit both you and the children you may have in the future.

SEEKING THE SELF

Seeking the self in the midst of all this stress and distress is probably the last thing you feel like doing. You would like some answers and a solution. You would like it to be over. You want to go on with your life.

Of course.

But somehow, no matter how soon we want it to be over, it's never over soon enough. And even when it's over, we carry it around with us. For many people, infertility never goes away completely. It was an issue for too long. An issue of enormous importance. The more that happens in our life and in the relationship while we wait for a solution, the more there remains to be sorted out.

In the broadest sense, resolving infertility is probably a lifelong process. No matter how brief or how long the struggle lasts, we somehow are never able to take life for granted again. We have learned that life doesn't move in a straight line, after all. We can't go blithely along anymore, expecting everything to turn out our way. And, having begun to question the meaning of life, we question ourselves—our purpose in life, our values, our lifestyle. Everything. Even if, in the end, we reconfirm everything about ourselves with which we started out, we have—in the process—changed.

Changes in identity are inevitable, for everyone, in every walk of life. What is more, they are healthy. When we consciouly seek to know ourselves better, to find ourselves and understand ourselves to the fullest, we capitalize on our potential to lead a rich life. The better we know ourselves, the more self-actualizing we become.

This process—of becoming more fully ourselves—often results from the force of circumstances, especially those circumstances we wish were not part of our life. We are "set up" for identity changes when we least want them or expect them. The choices we make in life revolve around our identity. We can take chances and plunge into something new and unknown, or we can trod the safest path. When we are in pain, following the straight and narrow seems easiest. But it's not necessarily the best thing for us to do.

Make the most of this opportunity in disguise to find yourself. You can be sure of one thing: Your life will change forever, in unknowable ways.

SEEKING THE SELF THROUGH RITUAL

Formal acknowledgment of this dislocation to your life and the pain you have endured may help you to break with the past—to incorporate this experience into your identity and move into the future. As I suggested in Chapter 8, there are no rituals to help mourn infertility or acknowledge its significance in our lives. A ritual of your own making may enable you to close this chapter of your life and go on. In *An Image Darkly Forming*, Bani Shorter describes the rituals five different women created for themselves to punctuate their passage through a life transition and to acknowledge its importance in their life.

The ritual you create is of your own making—it can be *anything* you devise. Your ritual could be intensely private—a one-person healing ceremony involving only you. Around the world, rituals have many ingredients—a trek to a sacred place, eating special food, changing into new or unusual clothes, adorning oneself in a different manner. Rituals may involve flowers, prayer, music, meditation, the expression of many emotions, cleansing the body, or cleansing the mind through quiet contemplation.

Or you could involve your partner and together create a ritual that has meaning for you both. For example, if you and your partner have had a miscarriage, perhaps a symbolic "funeral" would help you—something tangible that would acknowledge the depth of your loss. But it is not necessary to have miscarried or otherwise lost a child to do this. The pregnancy that never happened is just as valid, and just as great a loss.

Rituals not only mark endings, they signify new beginnings. Perhaps your ritual might be to initiate the adoption process, take steps to begin a new career, or celebrate the belated arrival of a child.

SEEKING GENERATIVITY

You can begin finding the new person you have become by seeking your own sense of generativity—now. Consider talking to a person your age or younger than you are—not necessarily a child—about a subject you have experience with. This could be anything. It could mean, for example, explaining to people how you have dealt with your infertility so that they may benefit.

Whatever you choose to do—and the possibilities are endless—notice the feelings you have from sharing what you know with others. Or experience the creativity that you feel upon learning something new that benefits you alone, by putting it to work. You will feel replete, filled up. You will be reminded that you have value as a person.

This is generativity.

THE FUTURE OF THE RELATIONSHIP

What more can I say about the relationship? Try to look at this whole experience as an *opportunity*—to grow together, to set off in new directions as a couple, to rediscover the person you were so attracted to long ago, and to find out who that person is in the process of becoming.

Many people go through life together without the relationship getting stirred up—with no major challenges or opportunities for change to occur. It's *boring* when this happens. You may be thinking, "I would love a little boring right now." Maybe, but what about when you're 60 and embarking on yet another new stage of life together? Do you want to wait until then to discover more about your partner? Do you want to put off until then the exploration of new ideas? To deepen your relationship in unknown ways? By then, it may be too late—you may have closed your mind to anything new in the relationship. You may have drifted apart out of boredom or apathy—or anger. The relationships in our lives, especially the one with our partner, provide us with the greatest opportunities for growth and change as individuals. Otherwise, we plod along unchallenged, and maybe, unchanging. A static existence that keeps us a prisoner of ourselves.

But if we are open to it, there is always something new in the offing—in ourselves and in our relationship. People do change. They don't stay the same. The problem is, we tend to do most of our big changes in troubled times, when we feel less equipped to handle change gracefully, or gladly. This is what change is all about. Out of pain, out of disjointed events in our lives that went awry, out of unfulfilled expectations, change is created. New parts of our self are born. And through them emerge the tantalizing, yet scary, prospects for our relationship.

Being open to the possibilities—facing the unknown future and letting it into our lives—is what makes life exciting.

> I was married before, and we achieved a certain level of success. But we didn't redream what we were going to do next. The next thing in life didn't open up. We ran out of dreaming. We ran out of the passion of it. We didn't have the tools to get on a different level so that dreams could become a reality in our life.
>
> Sandra and I are in the process of redreaming our lives now. Creating, making plans. The feeling I have about what we are doing is, 'This is it. This is right.' I have a vision of what we are going to do. Sometimes it is there with intensity.
>
> —Tony

ABOUT THE RESEARCH

Anthropologists often study small communities of people who are bound together by bonds that run deep—such as shared language, identical ethnic origins, shared life experience, kinship, lifelong social relationships, and other cultural ties.* Whether they are studying a tribal village in Africa, a street gang in the United States, or a different sort of small community, such as a hospital unit, anthropologists rely to a considerable extent on exploring the *shared* aspects of the community in order to understand the cultural context in which people live their lives. To do this, anthropologists participate in group life, by living among the people, socializing with them, attending their rituals and their religious ceremonies, eating their food, talking with them.

And they listen. They listen while the people they study talk to each other, they listen to what is said, to how individuals themselves interpret the events in their lives and what they make of them. It is through these avenues that anthropologists come to understand the cultural meanings that people attach to their lives. All these activities are part of "participant-observation," the research process by which anthropologists participate in and observe the life of the people. This method, together with interviewing, is the anthropologist's traditional way of collecting information, or "data." This highly intensive mode of ethnographic research is exactly suited to the name given to it—"field work."

I am no exception to this tradition. I had immersed myself in a

*See Robert Redfield, *The Little Community*. Chicago: University of Chicago Press, 1953.

cultural setting and done participant-observation daily for months before conducting any interviews. For example, when I studied deafness, I learned sign language in order to communicate with people and in order to fit in. When I studied the experience of having a stroke, I "lived" a good part of each day on a rehabilitation unit. When I studied homeless and socially marginal youth, I "hung out" in a transient neighborhood.

Now that I was going to study infertility, there was nowhere to hang out. I was apprehensive about only doing interviews, without being literally grounded by the cornerstone of my trade. Not only that, I was planning to study my own culture and cultural niche—something anthropologists have seldom done, until recently. To top it all off, I was going to study *myself*—people like me, in the same stage of life as I was, with the same goals and values, with the same health problem—people who carried with them a scenario for their lives similar to my own.

The question I was faced with—how so much sameness might affect my objectivity and my ability to gain insight—loomed large. To make matters even more complicated, as a graduate student I had repeatedly been warned, "Don't study yourself!" This voice, in stentorian tones, echoed in my head as I planned the research.

Considerable soul-searching followed as I asked myself whether I could effectively do what I intended. To help me gain clarity, I talked with other social scientists who had studied their own problem. I sounded out physicians I knew, who knew me and my work, about the feasibility of the study. I interviewed infertility specialists about what they considered to be the critical issues. I tried out my ideas on friends, who responded enthusiastically and went on to make suggestions.

Unlike some of my enthusiasms that ignite, only to quickly peter out, I found that not only was my excitement growing daily, I was already collecting data! I began the research, reassured by a grant from the Academic Senate of the University of California, San Francisco, that this was a viable—even legitimate—research project. Robert Nachtigall became my research partner.

I collected data from forty-three couples in two stages. During a one-and-a-half-year period in 1984–1985, I interviewed twenty-eight couples. These couples volunteered after hearing about the study from infertility specialists I had talked with, or they were recruited by persons already in the study. At the end of each interview, I always asked a couple if they would tell others they knew that I was looking for volunteers. (This method of locating respondents is known as the "snowball sampling technique.")

In 1987, while analyzing the data, I decided to do some additional interviews. I was working full-time on other research, as I had been during the first "wave" of interviewing, so I had some trepidation about the deluge that might ensue when I placed a request for volunteers in a Resolve newsletter. I worried needlessly that more people might respond than I could find the time to talk with. Reminded again that infertility is hard to talk about, I interviewed an additional eight couples and seven women, who chose to be interviewed without their partners. Although I had gone back several times to interview men and women separately in the first wave of interviewing, I conducted only one joint interview with most of the couples I talked with in 1987.

Volunteers for the research were spread throughout a broad geographic area. I visited couples by appointment, usually when they were home in the evening. I would jump in my car and drive long distances, reviewing what I knew about them. What had they told me on the phone? Were they in the midst of a particular crisis? Had they described a particular turning point that had made talking with me easier? Sometimes couples felt ready to talk because they thought they were in the process of resolving their infertility. Had they indicated that when we first talked?

This part of my field work was very familiar—reminiscent of working in a small, cohesive community—as I picked up the threads from the previous contact and moved on to develop them. By the time I arrived at their home, my mind emptied of other subjects, I felt as if I had never left the research for a minute, that my focus on infertility was total.

This single-minded approach to research is critical so that the researcher never loses touch with the subject at hand. Keeping the many new insights that arise in the course of the research carefully balanced in her head, she moves into the research encounter like a waiter, arms tiered with entrees, who glides into the restaurant to serve three tables at once. And, like a waiter, she is prepared to field falling plates, handle special orders, and repair any damage that is done.

Some anthropologists handle this tall order with dignity and aplomb. Unruffled, they can stay awake for three-day curing ceremonies, or, at least, outlast their informants. Not me. With the ever-present specter in my mind of how I slept, exhausted, on a bus coming home from Reno, while my deaf informants talked and told jokes—no doubt divulging the entire contents of their culture while I slept—it was with foreboding that I prepared each time to rise to the challenge.

I arrived, invariably somewhat disheveled, juggling my tape recorder, several tapes, and a handful of consent forms about participation in the research. At the door I was faced with the unknown. What kind of welcome would I receive? Sometimes people were nervous, sometimes they were smiling, sometimes they had forgotten I was coming. And occasionally there was only an empty house.

But once I was there and they invited me in, I forgot everything else. They had my rapt attention. I forgot I was tired, I forgot time, I forgot where I was, so involved did I become in what unfolded. Sometimes I forgot to stop and let them go to bed. Nobody seemed to notice.

The interview began as I explained the confidential nature of the research, what I would do with the information, and how I would keep it confidential. Couples were always very interested in all the details. They often asked a number of questions to learn how I would protect their identity. In research on other topics, whenever I brought out consent forms and began talking about confidentiality, people often waved the forms away with statements such as, "It doesn't matter—I'll sign anything," or "My life is an open book." This was not the case for persons living with infertility, reminding me each time anew that infertility is an intensely private matter.

Once we had discussed the protection of their anonymity to their satisfaction, I began the interview, often with the statement that I would try not to take up too much time. Couples, suddenly looking alarmed that this process would not quickly be over, became tense as I turned on my tape recorder and began asking questions from the interview guide.

My first question was global and intended to both break the tension and learn all about them: "Tell me everything that has happened since you first decided to have children." Couples quickly became caught up in their story that had altered their personal history and relationship forever. They began to recount the events of the preceding months and years. They hardly appeared to notice after the first few minutes that they were being interviewed. I kept asking questions and replacing tapes, and the hours flew by, while they, reliving again this painful period of their life, told me—and each other—their thoughts, feelings, and experiences amidst tears and laughter, disagreements, demonstrations of closeness, and expressions of love.

The resulting transcripts provide some of the richest data I have ever collected, and certainly the most rewarding. Only a fraction of what I learned from these wise and forthright men and women appears in this ethnography (the anthropologist's word for the study of a group of people).

A thumbnail sketch of the couples in the research shows them to be a cross-section of the population social scientists refer to as "middle Americans." They were predominantly white. Only two were black and one was Chinese. Their religious backgrounds were Protestant, Jewish, and Catholic, although the majority of respondents were not actively religious.

These women and men were employed primarily in professional and white-collar work. They were college educated almost without exception, and some had advanced degrees. Men's occupations included lawyer, writer, banker, psychologist, architect, and computer programmer, while women's occupations included teacher, social worker, business administrator, nurse, secretary, and designer. Three quarters of the couples owned their own homes.

Almost all in the study were in their thirties and forties. The youngest men and women were 28 and the oldest were 45 and 46. The average age of women and men was 36 and 37, respectively. Most had not attempted to conceive until the age of 30 or later. Almost all the couples were in infertility treatment at the time they were interviewed.

At the time they sought infertility treatment, five couples had one living child, and the remainder had none. The majority of couples had experienced infertility for two or more years. There were only four persons who had tried to conceive for less than two years. Nineteen couples had been in an infertility work-up for two or three years, and twenty couples had been in infertility treatment for four years or more. Their long-term experience of infertility may have influenced their willingness to talk to me.

After the interviews were completed, I would occasionally hear from couples about their "progress." Twenty couples recontacted me by mail: thirteen to say they had conceived and had a child, and seven couples to say they had adopted. I also heard from several couples who reported they were planning at the time to remain childless, but the final vote wasn't in. That's what Roger and I did.

I conducted what anthropologists call a "qualitative content analysis" on the data. I began by looking at the relationship between gender and infertility factor, and then at the actual words people used to describe themselves and their infertility. I looked carefully at who said what, and how women and men framed their responses to questions. As the data analysis proceeded, the questions that I asked in analysis became finer grained and delved deeply into each topic in the interview guide.

Throughout this process, I was concerned with letting the interpretations emerge that men and women placed on the events in their lives, not to alter their meanings to fit my own unconscious agenda. The possibility of imposing one's own truths and beliefs on the data is a risk that every social scientist lives with, no matter how research is conducted—whether through the collection of "facts" and numbers, or through the "softer" process of analyzing and interpreting life experiences. The way that research questions are formed and their translation into interview questions affects this process. Only time, and more research on this subject, will tell if I have accurately portrayed the effects of infertility on a couple's relationship.

By the time I completed the research, the issue of being unable to conduct research with a small cultural group, where I could observe "culture" at first hand through their interactions with each other, had long been forgotten. Indeed, it seemed that, for all the differences I did discover—in value orientations, underlying religious beliefs, and life plans—the persons in this study, and others like them who experience unwanted childlessness, did form part of a "little community," bound together by one common thread—their infertility.

One day I was sitting in the audience at a Resolve symposium and saw two women who had participated in the research sitting side by side, talking to each other animatedly. I did a double take. I didn't know they knew each other, but they were talking like old friends. As I approached them, they each saw me and headed my way. But, as it turned out, they had never met each other before, nor were they connected by any network of friends in the sample.

They were simply two women who came together for a brief moment in time. Two women who shared a common bond.

EPILOGUE

WRITING POPULAR ETHNOGRAPHY

In 1991, the year after *Healing the Infertile Family* was first published, anthropologist Karen Pliskin organized a session, "Going Public," for the Annual Meeting of the American Anthropological Association. She invited anthropologists who were known for their work in communicating anthropology to the general public to give papers, and she included me.[1] The American Anthropological Association had already given attention to this topic in their Newsletter, and because they believed it was important, they gave the session special status, designating it as "invited," publicizing it, and assigning the session to a ballroom in prime time. I was excited. Maybe the time had come at last when anthropologists would turn their attention to communicating with the public. But my hope was premature. The turnout was small. The Association gave a recap of the session in its Newsletter to call further attention to the topic. There was little response. Dismayed by the complete disinterest shown by most anthropologists in communicating with the public, I turned my energies to writing up my work for academic journals and carried on with my research. As I pursued the more academic aspects of my work, I wondered if the discipline of anthropology would *ever* consider it important to communicate with the public.

Although psychology, sociology, political science, economics, and history have come to the fore in informing presidents and publics on a sweeping range of issues, anthropology continues to be viewed by the public as romantic and irrelevant to everyday life. As a discipline that is grounded in the academy, anthropology gives few rewards to its practitioners who popularize their work. The lack of interest shown by most anthropologists in communicating with the general public is not new, however. Margaret Mead, the best known popularizer of anthropology, was ignored or not taken seriously by many of her peers. She was a controversial figure throughout her career; her discipline responded to her with ambivalence and sometimes with embarrassment despite the success with which she brought anthropology into the public domain.[2]

Today, a new generation of voices has emerged, to practice popular anthropology and to argue for its importance. In Great Britain and the United States a handful of anthropologists has traced the efforts of anthropologists, historically, to communicate beyond disciplinary boundaries, and recorded the ambivalence and distaste with which these efforts have been met in the academy.[3] The emphasis in academic anthropology is on making theoretical advances and on teasing out a topic in all its complexity rather than on simplifying or explaining it in a straightforward manner. Making work accessible to non-academics is the antithesis of this approach. Jeremy MacClancy, referring to this as cultural snobbism, observes that anthropologists are supposed to examine ideologies rather than reproduce them.[4]

Anthropology's traditional role has been to demonstrate, usually through cross-cultural comparisons, that taken-for-granted ideas in a given society are cultural rather than "natural." The cultural relativism embedded in anthropology creates a tendency to critique culture and challenge cherished cultural assumptions that people hold. Work categorized as popular anthropology has been dismissed on two counts—as failing to be critical and as reproducing the status quo. The primary danger of popularizing anthropological work lies in the potential that the status quo may be reaffirmed rather than questioned. Popularizing anthropology may be seen as a threat to the discipline of anthropology by undermining the work anthropologists have viewed as their primary task.

It is not surprising that there are many academic writers of ethnography and few popular writers in anthropology. While one receives academic rewards and encouragement, the other does not. Popular ethnography poses a threat to identity and academic training. The reticence to speak to the public and apply what anthropologists know has several sources. First, popular ethnography may appear unscholarly. Second, writing for the general public may appear to reduce cultural significance to something concrete. Third, many anthropologists continue to find validation, if not employment, in the academy. Fourth, anthropologists' need to be somehow different from those they study reaffirms the view of the anthropological self as "in between" cultures or as an observer of cultures. When anthropologists choose to write for the lay public, they must grapple with these issues.

TEARING DOWN BOUNDARIES

Recent developments in anthropology have the potential to reshape the acceptability of popular anthropology to academic anthropologists as well as the way popular anthropology is viewed by the public. The turn to experimental ethnography in the 1980s, while grounded in the academy and viewed by some as fostering greater elitism,[5] has inadvertently set the stage for the increased acceptability of popular ethnography. Experimental ethnography has been very influential in current anthropological writing, and consequently, its constraints affect all others, suggesting that ethnographic writing in general needs to be rethought. Experimental ethnography has been a primary expression of postmodernism in anthropology. The critique of ethnography initiated in the mid-1980s by anthropologists such as James Clifford, George Marcus, and Michael Fischer generated an explosion of ethnographic writing.[6] Those writers problematize ethnography by exploring relationships between ethnography and "science" and between ethnography and literature. They call for plural texts that engage multiple voices, heightened reflexivity, greater self-consciousness on the part of authors, and the use of the text to undermine the status quo. Experimental ethnography, as defined by these writers, is characterized by a cross-cultural focus, an emphasis on the writing process itself, and a meaning-centered approach to the topic.

Experimental ethnography has torn down boundaries in ethnographic writing, resulting in a proliferation of all kinds of ethnographic writing, not simply work that is defined as experimental. But by defining experimental ethnography as an intellectual endeavor of limited scope, questions have been raised about the place and worth of ethnographic writing that does not fit within academic bounds. Despite its many positive effects in transforming ethnography, experimental ethnography has also had the effect of promoting academic conceits. The delineation of experimental ethnography not only signaled a great creative advance, it perpetuated an exclusionary approach. One set of reigning hegemonies in anthropology was replaced with another.[7]

Experimental ethnography has been critiqued, in turn, for its omissions, especially with respect to popular texts and the work of women.[8] Jeremy MacClancy observes that, when experimental ethnographers critiqued classic texts, the renowned texts by which the discipline is known beyond its boundaries were completely overlooked. He points out that popular texts are still constructed texts that test the relationship between anthropology and literature.[9] Meanwhile, feminist anthropologists have responded with vigor to the comments James Clifford made in the Introduction to *Writing Culture* about why women anthropologists were not included in that volume.[10] The exclusion of feminist anthropologists has had the effect of provoking not only a further outpouring of important work but an increased determination to examine the many ways in which women in anthropology have contributed to the process of "writing culture," especially through the relationship between ethnography and literature. In doing so, feminist anthropologists have refused to separate creative and "critical" writing.[11] The refusal to set boundaries around what can be called critical writing or to limit critical writing to certain writing forms, combined with the willingness to experiment with all sorts of creative forms breaks apart, once and for all, traditional notions of what can be considered legitimate ethnography.

Feminist ethnography and popular ethnography are not necessarily equivalent, but the willingness of feminists to explore new writing modalities, as well as the rich heritage of women anthropologists, bodes well for the recognition of popular ethnography as a valuable genre that anthropologists can effectively utilize. Although women anthropologists do many kinds of writing,[12] popular ethnography aimed at the general public is seldom mentioned in the academic literature. The majority of popularizers in anthropology have been women in the United States and Great Britain. Judith Okely traces the popular writing of women anthropologists and observes that women have become popularizers because of interest in women's issues among the general public and because of their own marginalization in academic institutions.[13] This history has the effect of validating and further reinforcing the development of writing by feminist anthropologists. For example, although Mead's work aroused little interest among feminists except for a brief time in the 1960s,[14] now that there is a resurgence of interest in women anthropologists' writings, the works of Mead and many other women anthropologists are being revisited.

The removal of boundaries in ethnography by feminist anthropologists is a harbinger of things to come. Innovations often begin on the margins of a field and advance to its core. Like other innovations that have been initiated by feminist anthropologists and influenced anthropological thinking more broadly, this particular effort has the potential to spread across the discipline, undermine existing boundaries, and, in the process, make room for popular ethnography.

WRITING ETHNOGRAPHY FOR THE GENERAL PUBLIC

When I first decided to write a research-based book on infertility for the general public, I had not yet begun my research. I made this decision because little had been available to me to help me interpret my own experience when I underwent treatment for infertility. Many of the people I interviewed thought of themselves as veterans of infertility. They, too, wanted to see more information made available to people undergoing this experience. In writing *Healing the Infertile Family,* it was by far more important to me to reach the general public than to reach my academic peers.

This decision ultimately set off a struggle in me between my various identities: as a woman, as someone who had experienced infertility, as an anthropologist, and as an academic. While I was writing the book I had few doubts. It was only afterwards, when it was ignored by my fellow academics, that I came face to face with the full implications of writing popular ethnography in anthropology: the erasure of one's work by one's peers.[15] When core identities such as woman and anthropologist are assaulted by this sort of erasure, it provokes a radical rethinking of one's assumptions and actions. In my case, it deepened my commitment to popular ethnography, and, at the same time, forced me to look at my work anew. Asking myself what I had done and whether I still believed in doing it that way, I was compelled to reanalyze my text.

As I experimented with writing for the general public, I found the writing considerations were numerous. *Healing the Infertile Family* was written to fill a gap in the general public's knowledge about infertility and, at the same time, to address the issues that women and men undergoing infertility faced, both for their identity and their relationship with their partner. As such, it fits into Okely's category of women popularizing women's issues. But I also sought to do more than this: I wanted to bring anthropology to the public and to do it in a way that was reflexive. I wanted to demonstrate how anthropology can help people to make sense of their world and locate new meaning when what is meaningful has been lost. By showing my own engagement with the topic and the people I studied, and by illustrating the diversity of voices and approaches to the problem that I encountered in my research, I sought to bring anthropology to daily life. I wanted to show that anthropology is useful for more than an exotic look at faraway places. In doing so, I engaged concerns from experimental ethnography, feminist ethnography, and popular anthropology.

Issues about studying myself and using the "voices" of my respondents were engaged before the research began. Those issues have since become important in anthropology debates. Issues of voice have the same complexity in popular ethnography as in writing that is characterized as experimental ethnography. In the latter type of ethnographic writing, writers ponder at length the relationship between the anthropological self and others in order to reveal multiple voices. That writing is marked by writers' self-conscious attention to their own voices amid those of their respondents. Utilizing multiple voices is a tool that can be adapted for popular ethnography. For *Healing the Infertile Family,* I consciously made my own voice part of the book. I wrote myself into the preface and epilogue, as well as into the body of the book through the use of "we." In a book such as this, aligning oneself with one's readers is essential in order to empower people through shared experience and advocacy.

In taking on this task I incorporated cultural explanations only to the degree I thought they would be useful to people. I purposely did not write a cultural analysis, the term anthropologists use to refer to their analysis of the various components of a culture they are studying. Such analyses challenge the status quo by dissecting widely shared cultural assumptions. People who have experienced infertility have already had many of their cultural assumptions shattered, and when I wrote this book I believed that questioning cultural assumptions would not reaffirm people's sense of worth, which was my first goal. Rather I thought critical analysis would intensify the loss of meaning they experienced. I wanted to give readers the tools to work out personal solutions but I realized that only those solutions that adhered to their accepted cultural values would be meaningful.

In the intervening years since this book first appeared, I have changed my mind about the extent to which the assumptions people hold sacred can be challenged. By focusing only on individual change in *Healing the Infertile Family,* I became aware of the limitations of such an approach. At the same time, focusing on individual change sharpened my awareness of the role of culture. I repeatedly heard people in my research voice common cultural assumptions in the United States. Those assumptions shape how we respond to crises in our lives, such as infertility. Although I used to think challenging people's assumptions was dangerous when they were facing a crisis because of the possible loss of meaning they might experience, I now believe that this is precisely the moment in time that old assumptions can be challenged and that doing so may give people the courage to explore alternative ways to view their situation and seek action.

Like other kinds of ethnography, popular ethnography may express a particular point of view. Throughout this book I have tried to show how participating in a social group with similar concerns can be beneficial. In the course of doing research on infertility over the past fifteen years, I have repeatedly observed how being part of collective action can be a positive force in people's lives. Collective action can bring social change. The infertility self-help movement is an excellent example of this phenomenon. Fifteen years ago there was little acknowledgment of infertility in the media. Couples had few options—either medical or non-medical. Today, infertility is a recognized social problem in the United States. Industries have grown up around infertility—reproductive technologies and adoption—that need to be closely monitored. Although participation in collective action is not for everyone, for many people this kind of action can assuage a sense of difference and isolation from others, as well as foster social change. Not only are the effects of collective action potentially therapeutic, collective action constitutes an important means of undermining the status quo.

THE SECOND STUDY

The study that followed completion of the original edition of this book was more complex, thanks to funding from the National Institute on Aging. This time there were six interviewers. We carried out a study with 134 couples and 9 women without their partners who were either undergoing medical treatment at the time of the first interview or had completed medical treatment during the preceding three years. The majority had undergone medical treatment for three or more years, although 20 persons had undergone medical treatment for a year or less. Respondents were recruited from four sources: 1) 42 percent volunteered after seeing a printed flyer placed in physicians' private practices, HMOs, and low-income clinics; 2) 26 percent responded to a request for volunteers that appeared in a Resolve newsletter or flyer at Resolve workshops (a self-help organization for persons with infertility problems); 3) 25 percent were recruited by persons already in the study; and 4) 7 percent volunteered after hearing about the study from an adoption counseling service.

Demographic characteristics are available for 118 couples. The majority of respondents live in an urban or suburban area but 44 persons lived in rural areas. The age range for women was 26–52 (M = 36.13). For men the age range was 27–71 (M = 38.04). The sample was predominantly middle class and college educated, in a geographic locale that has one of the highest cost-of-living levels in the United States. The majority had yearly family incomes of $60,000 or more and owned their own homes; but 35 couples had family incomes below $60,000, and 4 families had incomes below $20,000. Eighty percent of couples had some form of health insurance, but less than half of those who were insured had any coverage for the medical treatment of infertility. Respondents were primarily in professional, management, and white collar employment; 97 women were employed outside the home and 21 were not employed; 114 men were employed and 4 were not employed. Forty persons (15 percent of the sample) were nonwhite or Latino (4 Native Americans, 14 Asian Americans, 12 African Americans, 6 Latinos, 2 East Indians, and 2 Pacific Islanders). With regard to religion, 43 were Catholic, 48 were Jewish, 55 were Protestant, 35 were members of other religions, 40 reported they had no religion, and 15 did not respond.

Partners were first interviewed together in detailed interviews lasting two hours or more; follow-up individual interviews took place approximately 6 to 12 months later, with final follow-up interviews with both partners taking place 12 to 24 months later. All interviews were audiotaped. We conducted interviews in English, with the exception of interviews with one couple in Spanish. Interviews addressed the events that led up to medical treatment, each person's experience of infertility, feelings, and related experiences, such as familial and work-related changes. To study the process that people undergo after infertility is discovered, we included closed- and open-ended questions, so that respondents could describe their experience in their own words. The exact wording of each question and the sequence of the questions was decided in the interview setting so that questions were relevant, tactful and appropriate for each situation. Interviewers used probes to elicit specific information about emotional reactions to infertility, attitudes about adoption, and effect of infertility on the marital relationship, and related topics. Interviews were taped and transcribed verbatim.

The data analysis for the second study followed the same overall approach as in the first study. The development of core categories was the first step in data analysis. A core category not only reappears often but also is continually analyzed for its implications for theory, its room for variation, and its linkages with other emergent core categories.[16] Core and emergent categories are developed through ongoing reading and analysis of transcripts and development of codes. Coding categories are generated from meanings inherent in the data themselves.[17]

Paradigm cases were used to develop the analysis in terms of range and variation in the data.[18] A paradigm case is a case that is a strong instance of something, that appears to be prototypical in the early stages of data analysis, before it can be categorized. A case-by-case analysis was carried out as well. The process begins with a close reading of each case for (1) repetition of specific words, phrases, and general thought patterns, (2) the structure of the overall case, and (3) the topics that dominated respondents' reports as well as topics that were not raised at all.[19]

NOTES

Identity and Fertility

Page 2. What it means to be a man or a woman.

Gender is not only biological, it is "cultural." Ortner and Whitehead, in *Sexual Meanings*, suggest that gender is a cultural idea that shapes individual behavior. Each society takes the biological differences of male and female and creates masculine and feminine identities, constructing culture-specific gender ideas that are rooted in a society's structures. Gender identity thus plays a critical role in the individual's definition of self.

Page 3. Definition of fertility.

Webster's New World Dictionary of the American Language, p. 516.

Page 4. Fertility in women starts to decline.

Federation CECOS, "Female Fecundity as a Function of Age," Office of Technology Assessment, *Infertility*, p. 52.

Page 4. Not much is known about male fertility.

Much less is known about male than female reproductive physiology, and consequently, methods to treat male infertility are underdeveloped. Office of Technology Assessment, *Infertility*, p. 107.

Page 4. The second is culture.

The term *culture* is used by anthropologists to refer to the system of meaning by which people interpret their own behavior and that of others (Spradley and McCurdy, *Conformity and Conflict*, p. 3). The concept of culture is broad and encompasses a multitude of ways of thinking that shape behavior, such as values, customs, manners, and beliefs. Geertz, in *Interpretation of Cultures*, says of the idea of culture, "Man is an animal suspended in webs of significance he himself has spun. I take culture to be those webs." (p. 5.) Culture is about meaning.

Page 5. The way we are raised leaves its imprint.

Socialization begins when a child is born and continues throughout life. It is through socialization—what we learn from other humans—that we become cultural beings capable of functioning in our society. Hallowell, *Culture and Experience*.

Page 10. Parenthood is a pivotal stage of the life cycle.

Gutmann, "Parenthood."

Page 10. Erikson calls this "generativity."

Erikson, *Childhood and Society*.

Page 10. There are other ways to nurture.

Daniels and Weingarten, *Sooner or Later*.

Page 13. Men may not think much about having a family.

Based on her research on childbearing and intentional childlessness, Kathleen Gerson, in *Hard Choices*, found that both men and women vary in their wish to bear children and their reasons for doing so, and concluded that men's and women's parenting motivations interact.

Page 14. Primary responsibility for the family life cycle.

Notman, "Changing Roles for Women in Mid-Life," p. 90.

Page 20. Parenting is a re-creation of oneself.

Hoffman and Manis, "The Value of Children in the United States."

Page 21. Parents turn to them for help.

Miller, *The Drama of the Gifted Child*.

Page 22. Repeating the past to get it right.

Lynda Schmidt, personal communication.

Trying

Page 28. Preparations gather steam.

Social scientists call the period of preparation for the next stage of life "anticipatory socialization," in which we rehearse new roles and emotionally adjust to life changes. Pearlin, "Discontinuities in the Study of Aging."

Page 36. Men and women lose their sense of motion through time.

Carter and McGoldrick, in *The Family Life Cycle*, describe how the interruption to the rhythm of movement through time can create an unexpected life transition and plunge a family into crisis at any stage of the family life cycle, (p. 5).

Identity Disruption

Page 39. The assumptions around which they have structured their lives.

Murray Parkes, "Psycho-social Transitions." Mathews and Mathews discuss the specific transition infertility initiates in "Infertility and Involuntary Childlessness."

Page 40. This inner world is our identity.

Becker, *Growing Old in Silence*, p. 39.

Page 40. They are in a crisis.

The crisis is provoked by the discontinuity in the life course. George, "Models of Transitions in Middle and Later Life."

Page 50. "Barren . . ."

Webster's Dictionary, p. 115.

Page 50. The ability to nurture others.

See Carol Gilligan, *In a Different Voice*, for an in-depth discussion of how women are socialized to nurture, and its effect on the self. In *The Pregnant Virgin*, Marion Woodman discusses the many meanings women attach to their bodies and the related roles they live out.

Page 50. Ideas of women as nurturers span a millennium.

Bolen, *Goddesses in Everywoman*; Teubal, *Sarah the Priestess*. See Becker, *Disrupted Lives*, on infertility and the body.

Page 52. Her body may have seemed like a machine.

The metaphor of the body as a machine is several centuries old. It has been suggested that the idea of the body as a machine continues to dominate medical practice, and affects how women, in turn, view their bodies. See Emily Martin's discussion in *The Woman in the Body*, chapter 4.

Page 53. "My body exploded."

Women who have ectopic pregnancies are at risk for the loss of an ovarian tube, serious illness, and even death. Ectopic pregnancies are on the rise in the United States, and quadrupled between 1970 and 1983 (Office of Technology Assessment, *Infertility*, p. 62). Both physicians and patients should be on the alert for this possibility when pregnancy occurs. In Marsha's case, her physician failed to correctly diagnose her symptoms, thus putting her life in jeopardy.

Page 57. She goes to the doctor.

Although one year of unprotected intercourse is the rule of thumb for seeking infertility treatment, women who are 35 or older or who have a medical history that suggests a problem may exist, such as DES or endometriosis, should not wait, nor should women who are extremely concerned about their fertility or that of their partner. Waiting under duress may load the emotional dynamics between partners because it reinforces men's reluctance to view the problem as real. Yet, seeking medical care is a trade-off. Couples face the possibility of being thrown headlong into an overmedicalized search for fertility, but, on the other hand, if they wait, they run the risk of dealing with the issue when time has truly run out. If a couple goes first to a gynecologist with a general practice, they should move on to an infertility specialist within six months of seeking medical treatment, if one is available in their community. Resolve's national headquarters keeps a nationwide list of infertility specialists.

Men and Identity

Page 59. He is some kind of cultural ideal.

Lederer, *The Fear of Women*. Zilbergeld, in *Male Sexuality*, debunks the stereotypes and expectations that surround male sexuality, and suggests a more down-to-earth model of sexuality for men and women to build on.

Page 60. A woman was seen as a passive receptacle.

From antiquity until the eighteenth century, women's bodies

were viewed as an inferior and inverted version of the male body (Laqueur, "Orgasm, Generation, and the Politics of Reproductive Biology," pp. 2–3). In some societies, the woman is viewed as having sole responsibility for fertility, and infertility is grounds for divorce. See Marcia Inhorn, *Infertility and Patriarchy; Quest for Conception.*

Page 61. The idea of male dominance.

Kimmel, "The Contemporary 'Crisis' of Masculinity," p. 122.

Page 61. A man's penis is at the center of his masculinity.

Monick, *Phallos*.

Page 61. Central to his sense of self.

See Zilbergeld, *Male Sexuality*; and Tiefer, "In Search of the Perfect Penis," for discussions of male sexuality.

Page 62. Men equate virility with potency.

In *Artificial Reproduction*, Snowdon and his colleagues suggest that men's inability to distinguish potency from fertility appears to place masculine self-esteem at greater jeopardy than infertility does for women. In interviews with sixty-six couples in England who underwent artificial insemination by donor, they found that the stigma attached to male infertility was viewed as much greater than that attached to female infertility.

Page 63. A man undergoes a complex emotional response.

Infertility, in general, has been discussed in terms of a stagelike response, similar to the adjustment process people go through for other life crises (see Menning, *Infertility*).

Page 65. They're not that straightforward.

Sperm have several major characteristics: their quantity, their motility, or ability to move toward the egg, their morphology—whether they are constructed in a certain way—and their ability to penetrate. Each of these characteristics is important to the viability of sperm. See Nachtigall and Mehren, *Overcoming Infertility*.

Page 66. There is little effective treatment for male infertility.

There *is* treatment for male infertility, including surgery and drug therapy, but success rates remain low. This field, medically termed "andrology," is growing, however, with concomitant increases in knowledge and treatment of male infertility. Some treatment modalities for male infertility are carried out on the female partner, such as artificial insemination by donor (DI) and in vitro fertilization (IVF), with varying rates of success. See Nachtigall and Mehren, *Overcoming Infertility*.

The Relationship

Page 75. "He thought it was just a problem of time and romance."

Research suggests that men are more romantic than women. Reedy in "Age and Sex Differences" found men to be more romantic than women. The usual sociological explanation is the power imbalance between women and men, and that women, because they have less power, are more realistic. In *Love in America*, Cancian suggests that men are more romantic because they are given less responsibility for working on the emotional relationship than women.

Page 76. When a man doesn't have a fertility problem.

The identity of men without a male infertility factor is less affected than men who have an infertility factor. Men without a male infertility factor usually do not describe themselves in terms of stigma nor do they report a stagelike response in adjustment to infertility. Nachtigall et al., "Effects of Gender-Specific Diagnosis."

Page 79. The sense of isolation a woman feels.

Social isolation is one of the commonly discussed experiences of women who are infertile. Bresnick and Taymor, in "The Role of Counseling in Infertility," found that women reported more isolation than men.

Page 81. They have fewer approved outlets for social exchange and intimacy.

Men may be less willing to *report* emotional closeness with other men than women are, but, even so, it appears that women have a greater number of close relationships than men (Cancian, *Love in America*, p. 75).

Page 81. Limits on a man's social self.

Clyde Franklin, in *The Changing Definition of Masculinity,* states that in adulthood men form many useful but superficial friendships with other men or with men who are mates of their partner's friends, thus facilitating "female dominance in expressive power." pp. 120–121.

Page 82. The myth says *real* men don't have failures.

Vittitow, in "Changing Men and Their Movement Toward Intimacy," cites as one of the ten commandments of manhood, "Thou shalt not fail."

Page 83. The idea that men are rational and women are emotional.

Studies show that Americans' role stereotypes for women include being illogical and the expression of tender feelings, while masculine qualities include being logical and hiding emotions (Broverman, "Sex Role Stereotypes and Clinical Judgments").

Page 84. According to our stereotypes about who does what.

Cancian, in *Love in America*, argues that in our culture love is feminized, which encourages women to be dependent and preoccupied with relationships, and men to be independent and preoccupied with work. She concludes that the feminization of love produces intense conflicts in marriage between women who want more closeness and men who withdraw (pp. 10–11). She suggests that part of the reason men *seem* so much less loving than women is that "men's behavior is measured with a feminine ruler," so men's expressions of love, such as practical help, spending time together, shared physical activities, and sex are disparaged in comparison with women's apparent superiority in intimate relationships.

Page 85. Alienation occurs.

Both Rubin, in *Intimate Strangers*, and Scarf, in *Intimate Partners*, describe polarized relationships and the rational/emotional dichotomy, while Sanford, in *The Invisible Partners*, discusses the underlying psychodynamics of this dilemma, pp. 35–41.

Page 88. "DI came up right from the beginning."

Donor insemination (DI) has been a commonly used treatment for male infertility for over forty years (Harkness, *The Infertility Book*, p. 203). For a discussion of the response of men and women during the years following their use of this procedure, see Snowden, *Artificial Reproduction*, which recounts research on the social and emotional experience of persons seen in one gynecologist's practice over a forty-year period in Great Britain. See Nachtigall and Mehren, *Overcoming Infertility*.

Page 90. Infertility invariably affects the sexual relationship.

Numerous authors have described the effect of infertility on the sexual relationship. See, for example, Menning, *Infertility*, and Seibel and Taymor, "Emotional Aspects of Infertility."

Page 92. A man funnels much of his emotional expression.

In *Love in America*, Cancian states that sexual intimacy is the only masculine way of expressing love that is culturally recognized in our society (p. 77).

Page 93. The regimentation and businesslike aura of this appointment.

In "Emotional Aspects of Infertility," Seibel and Taymor detail the way in which lovemaking becomes a test and partners experience difficulties in their sexual relationship—difficulties that reach their height during mid-cycle (p. 138).

Page 96. "It was a tremendous relief to both of us."

In artificial insemination by husband (AIH), the sperm are usually washed, by repeated centrifuging, from the protein and chemicals of the ejaculate before the insemination, and only a small amount of semen-free sperm are then inseminated into the uterus. Success rates range from 10 to 25 percent for intrauterine insemination, and 13 percent if the semen is inseminated into the vagina. Harkness, *The Infertility Book*, p. 204.

Facing the World

Page 100. We *do* feel different from others in a very specific way.

See Goffman, *Stigma*, for a discussion of the many facets of stigma.

Page 100. How women and men feel about themselves.

Descriptions of the stigma of infertility also appear in Miall, "The Stigma of Involuntary Childlessness," and in Snowden, *Artificial Reproduction.*

Page 104. Being part of an age group means we go through life in the same stages.

Social scientists call these age groups "cohorts." Whether we are "on time" or "off time" with the rest of our cohorts dramatically affects our views about whether we are moving through the life cycle as planned. Neugarten, "Adaptation and the Life Cycle."

Page 104. Friends anticipate the future together.

As friends go through life, they are socialized together to the next stage in life. Brim and Wheeler, *Socialization After Childhood.*

Page 104. Women are much more affected than men.

The research showed that women's relationships with other women were much more deeply affected than men's relationships with other men, which appeared to be affected little or not at all.

Page 105. Whatever it has always been still goes on, for them.

Socialization to parenthood appears to be a peripheral part of men's friendships, in contrast to women, for whom it is a central aspect of friendship at this time of life.

Page 106. The best friend's wife and baby.

The research found that while women's friendships may change when fertility becomes an issue, men's friendships only change if the partner experiences strain and conflict over their friends. In most cases where conflict arose, men's friendships continued, but sometimes in different social settings without their partners present.

Page 111. In adulthood we recognize our personal boundaries.

Fossum and Mason, in *Facing Shame*, discuss the development of personal boundaries and the interplay between privacy and shame within the family, pp. 59–83. Understanding these dynamics more fully may help to handle the public and private aspects of infertility.

Page 113. Like many other conditions that have stigma attached to them.

Becker and Arnold, "Stigma as a Social and Cultural Construct," pp. 51–54.

Family Matters

Page 128. Fathers don't usually enter into it much.

In her study of mother-daughter relationships, Fischer describes fathers as "outsiders." In all her families daughters grew up with greater intimacy with their mother than with their father. (*Linked Lives*, p. 18.)

Page 132. It's a script for Superwoman.

In "Beyond the Myth of Motherhood," Braverman analyzes the social and cultural components that contribute to the mother role.

Feelings

Page 138. Infertility is intangible.

Hertz calls infertility an "existential loss" in "Infertility and the Physician-Patient Relationship."

Page 139. No matter what the loss entails.

Judith Viorst, in *Necessary Losses*, discusses the many losses individuals sustain over the course of their lives and what the function of loss is for the individual.

Page 139. Grieving is essential.

Peter Marris, in *Loss and Change*, discusses the process of grieving and how, through grief, people create continuity for themselves.

Page 140. The hidden nature of infertility precludes public mourning.

In research with peoples all over the world, anthropologists have noted the importance of ritualized public mourning and its role in providing sustenance, support, and reinforcing life-affirming bonds with family and friends.

Page 140. Women go through a series of stages as they grieve.

A stagelike response has been described for the overall experience of infertility, as well as a stagelike response for grief. See Menning, "Emotional Needs of Infertile Couples."

Page 141. Denial enables women and men.

Menning, in "Emotional Needs," suggests that denial initially plays a necessary function in allowing individuals to adjust gradually to their infertility without shattering their identity.

Page 147. "I can't get to the point of adopting until I've grieved."

The research found that most women needed to go through a prolonged mourning period before they were ready to adopt. Mathews and Mathews, in "Infertility and Involuntary Childlessness," note that after adoption some women continue to pursue infertility treatment. This pattern was observed among women in both studies. These women all reported, however, that they were happy about the adoption, and that their investment in medical treatment and a biological child had greatly diminished.

Seeking Unity

Page 159. Assigning the disavowed parts of ourself.

An excellent discussion of projective identification can be found in Maggie Scarf's *Intimate Partners*, p. 62.

Page 159. A projection is hard to correct.

Von Franz, *Projections and Recollections*.

Page 164. Larry has distanced himself from the problem out of fear.

Steve Berman, in *The Six Demons of Love*, describes retreat as a common avoidance mechanism men employ in order to avoid examining their insecurities and to put the responsibility on their partner (pp. 55–56).

Working Together

Page 170. Family clinicians Carter and McGoldrick.

Developing Murray Bowen's idea of horizontal and vertical

stress, Carter and McGoldrick suggest that both types of stress go hand in hand with any unexpected life transition, in *The Family Life Cycle*, pp. 9–11.

Page 172. These values include achievement and success.

Anthropologists studying American populations repeatedly observe the effect of value orientations on people's lives. See Clark and Anderson, *Culture and Aging*; and Kaufman, *The Ageless Self*.

Page 175. The pattern partners develop together.

Kramer, *Family Interfaces*, pp. 3–33.

Page 175. They are often the only ones we know.

Fossum and Mason, in *Facing Shame*, describe how dysfunctional behavior is learned and repeats itself over the generations.

Page 176. When a woman excuses her partner.

Norwood, in *Women Who Love Too Much*, describes how women excuse their partner from active participation in the relationship.

Page 176. The potential for a deadlock to occur.

The other main pattern occurs when a man indicates he must have a child. Regardless of a woman's fertility status (i.e presence or absence of a fertility factor), she will feel like a failure, and their relationship may become polarized along a demand/failure to meet the demand continuum.

Page 178. If you are a woman protecting her man.

Discussions of this issue can be found in Norwood, *Women Who Love Too Much*, and in Kiley, *The Peter Pan Principle*.

Page 178. This dynamic eventually makes women wild with anger.

Several writers have addressed various aspects of this problem in relationships. See Mornell, *Passive Men, Wild Women*, for an overview that touches on some of the deeper issues.

Getting Help

Page 189. It has been found in clinical practice.

The importance of therapy services and sex counseling for

infertility has been repeatedly emphasized (Bresnick and Taymor, "The Role of Counseling in Infertility"; Menning, "Emotional Needs"; and Sarrel and DeCherney, "Psychotherapeutic Intervention for Treatment of Couples with Secondary Infertility").

Changes

Page 206. Applying for an in vitro fertilization program.

In vitro fertilization (IVF) programs used to have requirements that varied from one program to another. See Becker and Nachtigall, "'Born to Be a Mother'" for emotional risks related to IVF. Resolve is a clearinghouse for information on IVF programs.

Page 209. These symbols make sense out of the nonsensical.

Personal symbols reflect the subjective meaning we embue them with, and become a means to help in the interpretation of the events in one's life. Anthropologists have studied symbolic meaning cross-culturally, as a window through which to understand culture, while some schools of psychology, such as Jungian psychology, use cultural symbolism as a means to reach the deep self. See, for example, Geertz, *The Interpretation of Cultures*, and Jung, *Man and His Symbols*.

Page 211. Sooner or later we find the recognizable threads.

Marris, *Loss and Change*, pp 33–34.

Page 212. Continuity is *the* issue of mid-life.

Jung, in *Modern Man in Search of a Soul*, pp. 95–114, and Levinson, in *Seasons of a Man's Life*, have both suggested the process of self-integration begins in mid-life, perhaps as early as the thirties.

Page 215. It is what differentiates us from other species.

Humans are capable of expressing themselves and communicating in symbolic codes, such as language, games, and art forms. This capacity sets us apart from other species and enables us to develop unique interpretations about the nature of things. This is why humans are uniquely "cultural" beings. Symbolic forms and processes color our motivations and goals, our entire thinking and feeling life. Each of us interprets this symbolic system to create our own reality. (Hallowell, *Culture and Experience*, p. 7.)

Page 215. To develop the themes in our life story.

Kaufman, in *The Ageless Self*, illustrates how people develop themes that give rhyme and reason to their lives.

Page 215. It is because of memory that our life has continuity.

Neugarten, "Time, Age and the Life Cycle."

Page 216. She . . . was diagnosed as having endometriosis.

The effect of endometriosis on fertility varies among women. (Harkness, *The Infertility Book*, pp. 142–143.) For a complete discussion of endometriosis, see Older, *Endometriosis*.

Page 218. One of the tasks of mid-life is the restructuring of our values.

Samuels, *Jung and the Post-Jungians*, p. 102.

Page 218. We begin the individuation process.

Jung conceived the individuation process as the gradual realization of the self over a lifetime. That is, it is ongoing over the course of life and is never completed. Samuels, *Jung and the Post-Jungians*, pp. 101–102.

Remaking Roles

Page 227. Out of step with the timing of life stages.

Neugarten, "Adaptation and the Life Cycle."

Page 230. Cultural norms have historically dictated that women nurture, while men achieve.

Gilligan, *In a Different Voice*; Barnett and Baruch, "Women in the Middle Years."

Page 230. Cross-cultural studies of men and women in mid-life.

Gutmann, *Reclaimed Powers*.

Page 231. Carol Gilligan has suggested.

Gilligan, in *In a Different Voice*, has suggested that women are apparently more embedded in personal relationships than men are, and that they experience identity development differently as a result.

Page 232. This was true for women with highly successful careers.

Every woman in the research underwent a reassessment of her

nonparenting roles that involved self-expression. Searching for means of carrying out expressive roles provokes an intense process of inner searching, in which identity is redefined.

Page 234. Men who have a crisis in their career.

In contrast to the social pressures women experience against career achievement, men experience intense social pressures toward it. Because career success is such an important part of self-definition for men in mid-life, it should come as no surprise that all the men in the research who simultaneously underwent a career crisis and discovered they were infertile became temporarily overwhelmed by this dual blow to their manhood. In time, these men went on with their lives, but the adjustment process took time.

The Quest for Resolution

Page 237. Resolution is made up of many ingredients.

The process of reaching resolution has been discussed by various writers. See especially Menning, *Infertility*, pp. 104–117.

Reaching Resolution

Page 249. The nature and length of treatment.

It has been found that persons who have been in infertility treatment for two or more years reported becoming more circumspect about the lengths to which they would go in order to conceive. Individuals alter the way they attempt to control treatment—by limiting the amount of medical intervention they will tolerate, or by setting a time to terminate medical care. Many couples either identify a date or a procedure as a termination point for the infertility work-up. Others who plan to continue treatment alter their strategy to minimize its effect on daily life. Becker and Nachtigall, "Ambiguous Responsibility."

Page 252. Couples may remain out of step.

Men are ready to adopt long before women. Adoption may be more problematic for a woman than for a man because it removes the control over the pregnancy from her body. Women initially express concern over the many uncontrollable factors in the process, for example, the difficulty of finding a child, the possibility that the birth mother would wish to keep the child, and the child's genetic makeup. In contrast, men usually find adoption to be a viable solution to infertility and are in favor of it. They believe the pursuit of adoption will return control to a situation that may appear to be uncontrollable and increasingly hopeless.

Page 252. Adoption usually becomes more attractive to women.

In most cases, only when women have exhausted their medical options are they able to seriously consider adoption.

Page 252. Agency sponsored or private adoption.

Harkness, in *The Infertility Book*, provides an updated account of the differences between agency and independent adoption, and outlines the process leading up to undertaking adoption, pp. 217–233. Local Resolve chapters offer pre-adoption workshops that explore the process of adoption in detail.

Page 253. Sending out letters to various parts of the country.

Private adoption is legal in some states only. In *The Infertility Book*, Harkness describes the steps couples should take if they decide to undertake private adoption.

Page 256. It is men who balk at this possibility.

A man's decision to try artificial insemination by donor is usually arrived at only gradually, after a long and painful self-search. This option remains untenable for many men. Two thirds of the men in the research who were infertile chose not to try DI, although their partners indicated a willingness to try this method.

What Lies Ahead

Page 263. 20-minute rule.

Bombardieri, "The Twenty-Minute Rule."

Page 266. They *do* represent the norm.

Jean Veevers, in *Childless by Choice*, and Diana Burgwyn, in *Marriage Without Children*, both talk about what it means to be up against the norm for parenthood.

Page 267. It *shapes* our lives.

Geertz, in *Interpretation of Cultures*, sums up culture by saying, "Becoming human is becoming individual, and we become individual under the guidance of cultural patterns, historically created systems of meaning in terms of which we give form, order, point, and direction to our lives."(p. 52)

Page 273. Try to look at this whole experience.

Kast, in *The Nature of Loving*, states, "A tremendously stimulating aspect of love is its ability to allow us through fantasies to see ourselves anew and to grow beyond ourselves." (p. 6)

Page 273. The relationships in our lives.

In *The Invisible Partners*, Sanford discusses the intimate relationship and its potential for personal growth to occur (pp. 80–82), while Schmidt, in "The Brother-Sister Relationship in Marriage," views the intimate relationship as the arena in which both the self and the relationship can be developed to its fullest.

Notes to the Introduction

1. Gay Becker, *Disrupted Lives: How People Create Meaning in a Chaotic World.* (Berkeley: University of California Press, 1998).
2. Arthur L. Griel, T. A. Leitko, and Karen L. Porter, "Infertility: His and Hers," *Gender and Society* 2 (1988):172; Robert D. Nachtigall, Gay Becker, and Mark Wozny, "The Effects of Gender-Specific Diagnosis on Men's and Women's Response to Infertility." *Fertility and Sterility* 57 (1991): 113–121.
3. Charlene Miall, "The Stigma of Involuntary Childlessness," *Social Problems* 33 (1986): 268–282; Jean E. Veevers, "The Social Meanings of Parenthood," *Psychiatry* 36 (1973): 291–310.
4. For further discussions of the course of life as a cultural phenomenon, see: Christine L. Fry and Jennie Keith, "The Life Course as a Cultural Unit," In *Aging From Birth to Death.*

Vol. 2, Sociotemporal Perspectives, ed. Matilda White Riley, Ronald Abeles, and M.S. Teitelbaum. (Boulder, CO: Westview Press, 1982); Christine L. Fry, "The Life Course in Context: Implications of Comparative Research." In *Anthropology and Aging,* ed. Robert L. Rubinstein (Dordrecht, Netherlands: Kluwer, 1990), 129–49; John W. Meyer, "Levels of Analysis: The Life Course as a Cultural Construction," in *Social Structures and Human Lives,* ed. Matilda White Riley (Beverly Hills: Sage, 1988), 49–62; Robert L. Rubinstein, "Nature, Culture, Gender, Age," in *Anthropology and Aging,* ed. Robert L. Rubinstein, 109–15; Mark R. Luborsky, "The Romance with Personal Meaning in Gerontology: Cultural Aspects of Life Themes," *The Gerontologist* 33 (1993):445–52.

5. John W. Meyer, "Levels of Analysis"; Gay Becker, *Disrupted Lives.*
6. Gay Becker and Robert D. Nachtigall, "Eager for Medicalization: The Social Production of Infertility as a Disease," *Sociology of Health and Illness,* 14 (1992): 456–471.
7. Office of Technology Assessment, U. S. Congress, 1988. *Infertility: Medical and Social Choices* (Washington, D.C.: U.S. Government Printing Office, 1988).
8. Medicalization refers to the process by which human experiences are redefined as medical problems. See, for example, Eliot Friedson, *Profession of Medicine* (New York: Dodd Mead, 1970); Irving K. Zola, "Medicine as an Institution of Social Control;" *American Sociological Review* 20 (1972): 487–504.
9. Lois W. Hoffman and J. D. Vladis, "The Value of Children in the United States: A New Approach to the Study of Fertility." *Journal of Marriage and the Family* 41 (1979): 583–596.
10. R. Snowden, G. D. Mitchell, and E. M. Snowden, *Artificial Reproduction: A Social Investigation* (London: George Allen & Unwin, 1983).
11. Gay Becker and Robert D. Nachtigall, "Ambiguous Responsibility in the Doctor-Patient Relationship: The Case of Infertility." *Social Science and Medicine* 32 (1991): 875–885.

12. Becker and Nachtigall, "Eager for Medicalization."
13. David Schneider, *American Kinship: A Cultural Account,* 2nd Ed. (Chicago: University of Chicago Press, 1980).
14. For an illuminating look at how differently adoption is viewed in societies other than that of the United States, see John Terrell and Judith S. Modell, "Anthropology and Adoption," *American Anthropologist* 96 (1994), 155–161; for a cultural analysis of adoption in the United States, see Judith S. Modell, *Kinship with Strangers: Adoption and Interpretations of Kinship in American Culture* (Berkeley: University of California Press, 1994).
15. Gay Becker and Robert D. Nachtigall, "'Born to Be a Mother': The Cultural Construction of Risk in Infertility Treatment in the U.S." *Social Science and Medicine* 39 (1994): 507–518.
16. For other work on how couples' lives are affected by the use of reproductive technologies, see: Sarah Franklin, *Embodied Progress: A Cultural Account of Assisted Conception* (London: Routledge, 1997); Arthur L. Griel, *Not Yet Pregnant: Infertile Couples in Contemporary America* (New Brunswick, N.J.: Rutgers University Press, 1991); Margarete Sandelowski, *With Child in Mind: Studies of the Personal Encounter with Infertility* (Philadelphia: University of Pennsylvania Press, 1993).
17. Sylvia Yanagisako and Carol Delaney, "Naturalizing Power," in *Naturalizing Power: Essays in Feminist Analysis,* ed. Sylvia Yanagisako and Carol Delaney (New York: Routledge, 1995), 1–24.
18. Barbara Laslett and Johanna Brenner, "Gender and Social Reproduction: Historical Perspectives," *Annual Review of Sociology* 15 (1989): 381–404: 382.
19. Johanna Brenner and Barbara Laslett, "Social Reproduction and the Family." In *Sociology: from Crisis to Science? Vol. 2 The Social Reproduction of Organization and Culture,* ed. U. Himmenstrand (London: Sage, 1986), 116–31; Kath Weston, "Forever Is a Long Time: Romancing the Real in Gay Kinship Ideologies," In *Naturalizing Power,* 87–110.

20. For further details about these research findings, see Robert Nachtigall et al., "Effects of Gender-specific Diagnosis."
21. For a discussion of infertility as women's work and perceptions of risk among men and women, see Gay Becker and Robert D. Nachtigall, "'Born to Be a Mother.'"
22. Ibid.; Gay Becker and Robert D. Nachtigall, "'Selling Hope': Consumers' Shifting Views of New Reproductive Technologies," *Social Science and Medicine,* in press; Gay Becker, *The Elusive Embryo: Gender and Engagement with New Reproductive Technologies* (Berkeley: University of California Press, forthcoming).
23. See Gay Becker, *Disrupted Lives;* Gay Becker, "Metaphors in Disrupted Lives: Infertility and Cultural Constructions of Continuity," *Medical Anthropology Quarterly* 8 (1994): 383–410.

Notes to Epilogue

1. This discussion is based on a paper, "Popular Ethnography: Respectable and Scholarly?", presented at the American Anthropological Association Annual Meeting, November 1991.
2. Ruth Behar, "Introduction: Out of Exile," in *Women Writing Culture,* ed. Ruth Behar and Deborah A. Gordon. (Berkeley: University of California Press, 1995), 1–29; Nancy C. Lutkehaus, "Margaret Mead and the 'Rustling-of-the-Wind-in-the-Palm-Trees School' of Ethnographic Writing," in *Women Writing Culture,* 186–206; William E. Mitchell, "Communicating Culture: Margaret Mead and the Practice of Popular Anthropology," in *Popularizing Anthropology,* ed. Jeremy MacClancy and Chris McDonaugh. (London: Routledge, 1996), 122–134.
3. Jeremy MacClancy and Chris McDonaugh, eds. *Popularizing Anthropology,* (London: Routledge, 1996); Ruth Behar and Deborah A. Gordon, eds. *Women Writing Culture.* (Berkeley: University of California Press, 1995).

4. Jeremy MacClancy, "Popularizing Anthropology," in *Popularizing Anthropology,* 2.
5. Ibid., 2.
6. James Clifford and George E. Marcus, eds. *Writing Culture: The Poetics and Politics of Ethnography* (Berkeley: University of California Press, 1986); George E. Marcus and Michael M. J. Fischer, *Anthropology as Cultural Critique: An Experimental Moment in the Human Sciences* (Chicago: University of Chicago Press, 1986).
7. Jeremy MacClancy, "Popularizing Anthropology," in *Popularizing Anthropology,* 3.
8. Ibid.; Ruth Behar and Deborah A. Gordon, eds., *Women Writing Culture;* Margery Wolf, A *Thrice Told Tale: Feminism, Postmodernism, and Ethnographic Responsibility.* (Stanford: Stanford University Press, 1992).
9. Jeremy MacClancy, "Popularizing Anthropology," in *Popularizing Anthropology,* 3.
10. James Clifford, "Introduction," *Writing Culture;* see for example, Ruth Behar, "Introduction: Out of Exile," in *Women Writing Culture;* Deborah A. Gordon, "Writing Culture, Writing Feminism: The Poetics and Politics of Experimental Ethnography," Inscriptions 3/4 (1988): 8, 21; Margery Wolf, *Thrice Told Tale.*
11. See Ruth Behar and Deborah A. Gordon, eds., *Women Writing Culture;* Cherrie Moraga and Gloria Anzaldua, eds., *This Bridge Called My Back: Writings by Radical Women of Color* (New York: Kitchen Table, Women of Color Press, 1983).
12. Ibid.
13. Judith Okely, "Women Readers: Other Utopias and Own Bodily Knowledge," in *Popularizing Anthropology,* 180–207.
14. Ibid., 181.
15. In "The Erasure of Women's Writing in Sociocultural Anthropology," (*American Ethnologist* 17 (1990): 611–627), Catherine Lutz calls attention to how citation patterns in anthropology have "erased" the work of women anthropologists. It should be noted, however, that women anthropologists themselves participate in the erasure of women's work,

namely, popular anthropology in academia. Relevant popular anthropology works are seldom cited in academic work. This is all the more noticeable because much of that work is about women and is written by women. See Judith Okely, "Women Readers," in *Popularizing Anthropology.*

16. Carolyn Wiener, *The Politics of Alcoholism.* (New Brunswick, NJ: Transaction, 1981).
17. Elliott Mishler, *Research Interviewing.* (Cambridge: Harvard University Press, 1986).
18. Patricia Benner, *From Novice to Expert.* (Menlo Park, CA: Addison Wesley, 1984).
19. Sharon Kaufman, *The Ageless Self.* (Madison: University of Wisconsin Press, 1986).

BIBLIOGRAPHY

The Family and Parenting

Braverman, Lois. "Beyond the Myth of Motherhood." In Monica McGoldrick, Carol M. Anderson, and Froma Walsh, eds., *Women in Families: A Framework for Family Therapy*. New York: W. W. Norton, 1989, pp. 226–266.

Burgwyn, Diane. *Marriage Without Children*. New York: Harper & Row, 1981.

Carter, Elizabeth A. and Monica McGoldrick, eds. *The Family Life Cycle: A Framework of Family Therapy*. New York: Gardner Press, 1980.

Daniels, Pamela and Kathy Weingarten. *Sooner and Later: The Timing of Parenthood in Adult Lives*. New York: W. W. Norton, 1982.

Fischer, Lucy Rose. *Linked Lives: Adult Daughters and Their Mothers*. New York: Harper & Row, 1986.

Gerson, Kathleen. *Hard Choices*. Berkeley, CA: University of California Press, 1985.

Gutmann, David. "Parenthood: A Key to the Comparative Study of the Life Cycle." In Nancy Datan and Leon Ginsburg, eds., *Life-Span Development Psychology, Normative Life Crises*. New York: Academic Press, 1975.

Hoffman, Lois W. and Jean D. Manis. "The Value of Children in the United States: A New Approach to the Study of Fertility." *Journal of Marriage and the Family*, 41:583–596, 1979.

Kramer, Jeannette R. *Family Interfaces: Transgenerational Patterns*. New York: Brunner/Mazel, 1985.

Veevers, Jean E. "The Social Meanings of Parenthood." *Psychiatry*, 36:291–310, 1973.

———. *Childless by Choice*. Toronto: Butterworths, 1980.

Infertility and Related Issues

Becker, Gay and Robert D. Nachtigall. "Ambiguous Responsibility in the Doctor-Patient Relationship: The Case of Infertility." *Social Science & Medicine*: 32:875–85, 1991.

Becker, Gay and Robert D. Nachtigall. "'Born to Be a Mother': The Cultural Construction of Risk in Infertility Treatment." *Social Science & Medicine*: 39:507–518, 1994.

Bombardieri, Merle. "Child-free Decision-Making," a twelve-page reprint available from Resolve's national office.

———. "The Twenty-Minute Rule: First Aid for Couples in Distress." *Resolve National Newsletter*, 5, December, 1983.

Bresnick, Ellen and Melvin Taymor. "The Role of Counseling in Infertility." *Fertility and Sterility*, 32:154–156, 1979.

Federation CECOS, D. Schwartz, and M. J. Mayaux. "Female Fecundity as a Function of Age: Results of Artificial Insemination in 2193 Nulliparous Women with Azoospermic Husbands." *New England Journal of Medicine*, 306:404, 1982.

Fertility and Pregnancy Guide for DES Daughters and Sons. San Francisco: DES Action, USA, n.d.

Friedman, Rochelle and Bonnie Gradstein. *Surviving Pregnancy Loss*. Boston: Little, Brown, 1982.

Harkness, Carla. *The Infertility Book*. San Francisco: Volcano Press, 1987.

Hertz, Dan G. "Infertility and the Physician-Patient Relationship: A Biopsychosocial Challenge." *General Hospital Psychiatry*, 4:95–101, 1982.

Kraft, Adrienne D., Joseph Palombo, Dorena Mitchell, Catherine Dean, Steven Meyers, and Ann Wright Schmidt. "The Psychological Dimensions of Infertility." *American Journal of Orthopsychiatry*, 50:618–628, 1980.

Mathews, Ralph and Ann Mathews. "Infertility and Involuntary Childlessness: The Transition to Nonparenthood." *Journal of Marriage and the Family*, 48:641–649, 1986.

Menning, Barbara E. "Emotional Needs of Infertile Couples." *Fertility and Sterility*, 34:313–319, 1980.

——— *Infertility: A Guide for the Childless Couple*. Englewood Cliffs, NJ: Prentice-Hall, 1977.

Miall, Charlene. "The Stigma of Involuntary Childlessness." *Social Problems*, 33:268–282, 1986.

Nachtigall, Robert D. "Disorders of the Ovary and Female Reproduction." In Paul Fitzpatrick, ed., *Handbook of Clinical Endocrinology*. Greenbrae, CA: Jones Medical Publications, 1986.

Office of Technology Assessment, U.S. Congress. *Infertility: Social and Emotional Choices*. Washington, DC: Government Printing Office, 1988.

Older, Julia. *Endometriosis*. New York: Charles Scribner's Sons, 1984.

Sarrel, Philip M. and Alan H. DeCherney. "Psychotherapeutic Intervention for Treatment of Couples with Secondary Infertility." *Fertility and Sterility*, 43:897–900, 1985.

Seibel, Machelle M. and Marvin L. Taymor. "Emotional Aspects of Infertility." *Fertility and Sterility*, 37:137–145, 1982.

Snowden, R., G. D. Mitchell, and E. M. Snowden. *Artificial Reproduction: A Social Investigation*. London: George Allen & Unwin, 1983.

Gender

Barnett, Rosalind C. and Grace K. Baruch. "Women in the Middle Years: A Critique of Research and Theory." *Psychology of Women Quarterly*, 3:187–197, 1978.

Broverman, Inge, Donald Broverman, Frank Clarkson, Paul Rosenkrantz, and Susan Vogel. "Sex Role Stereotypes and Clinical Judgments of Mental Health." *Journal of Consulting Psychology*, 34:1–7, 1970.

Cancian, Francesca M. *Love in America: Gender and Self-Development*. New York: Cambridge University Press, 1987.

Franklin, Clyde W. *The Changing Definition of Masculinity*. New York: Plenum, 1984.

Gilligan, Carol. *In a Different Voice*. Cambridge, MA: Harvard University Press, 1982.

Guttman, David. *Reclaimed Powers: Toward a New Psychology of Men and Women in Later Life*. New York: Basic Books, 1988.

Kimmel, Michael S. "The Contemporary 'Crisis' of Masculinity in Historical Perspective." In Harry Brod, ed., *The Making of Masculinities: The New Men's Studies*. Boston: Allen and Unwin, 1987, pp. 121–154.

Laqueur, Thomas. "Orgasm, Generation, and the Politics of Reproductive Biology." In Catherine Gallagher and Thomas Laqueur, eds., *The Making of the Modern Body: Sexuality and Society in the Nineteenth Century*. Berkeley, CA: University of California Press, 1987, pp. 1–41.

Lederer, Wolfgang. *The Fear of Women*. New York: Harcourt Brace Jovanovich, 1968.

Martin, Emily. *The Woman in the Body: A Cultural Analysis of Reproduction*. Boston, MA: Beacon Press, 1987.

Monick, Eugene. *Phallos: Sacred Image of the Masculine*. Toronto: Inner City Books, 1987.

Notman, Malkah T. "Changing Roles for Women at Mid-Life." In William H. Norman and Thomas J. Scaramella, eds., *Mid-Life: Development and Clinical Issues*. New York: Brunner/Mazel, 1980, pp. 85–109.

Ortner, Sherry B. and Harriett Whitehead. *Sexual Meanings: The Cultural Construction of Gender and Sexuality*. Cambridge, MA: Cambridge University Press, 1981.

Reedy, Margaret N. "Age and Sex Differences in Personal Needs and the Nature of Love." Ph.D. dissertation, Department of Psychology, University of Southern California, 1977.

Teubal, Sarah J. *Sarah the Priestess: The First Matriarch of Genesis*. Athens, OH: Swallow Press, 1984.

Tiefer, Lenore. "In Search of the Perfect Penis: The Medicalization of Male Sexuality." In Michael S. Kimmel, ed., *New Directions in Research on Men and Masculinity*. Beverly Hills, CA: Sage Publications, 1987, pp. 165–184.

Vittitow, D. "Changing Men and Their Movement Toward Intimacy." In R. A. Lewis, ed., *Men in Difficult Times*. Englewood Cliffs, NJ: Prentice-Hall, 1981.

Zilbergeld, Bernie. *Male Sexuality*. Boston, MA: Little, Brown, 1978.

Relationships

Berman, Steve. *The Six Demons of Love*. New York: McGraw-Hill, 1984.

Kast, Verena. *The Nature of Loving: Patterns of Human Relationship*. Wilmette, IL: Chiron Publications, 1984.

Kiley, Dan. *The Peter Pan Principle: Men Who Have Never Grown Up*. New York: Dodd, Mead & Co., 1983.

Mornell, Pierre. *Passive Men, Wild Women*. New York: Ballantine, 1979.

Norwood, Robin. *Women Who Love Too Much: When You Keep Wishing and Hoping He'll Change*. New York: Simon & Schuster, 1985.

Rubin, Lillian. *Intimate Strangers*. New York: Harper & Row, 1983.

Sanford, John A. *The Invisible Partners*. New York: Paulist Press, 1980.

Scarf, Maggie. *Intimate Partners: Patterns in Love and Marriage*. New York: Random House, 1987.

Schmidt, Lynda W. "The Brother-Sister Relationship in Marriage." *Journal of the Society of Analytical Psychology*, 25:17–35, 1980.

Psychology and Self-Help

Bolen, Jean S. *Goddesses in Everywoman*. New York: Harper & Row, 1984.

Fossum, Merle and Marilyn Mason. *Facing Shame: Families in Recovery*. New York: W. W. Norton, 1986.

Jung, Carl, ed., *Man and His Symbols*. New York: Dell, 1968.

———. *Modern Man in Search of a Soul*. Translated by W. S. Dell and C. F. Baynes. New York: Harcourt Brace, 1933.

Miller, Alice. *The Drama of the Gifted Child*. New York: Basic Books, 1981.

Samuels, Andrew. *Jung and the Post-Jungians*. London: Routledge & Kegan Paul, 1985.

Shorter, Bani. *An Image Darkly Forming*. London: Routledge & Kegan Paul, 1987.

Viorst, Judith. *Necessary Losses*. New York: Fawcett, 1986.

Von Franz, Marie Louise. *Projections and Recollections in Jungian Psychology: Reflections of the Soul*. London: Open Court, 1980.

Woodman, Marion. *The Pregnant Virgin: A Process of Psychological Transformation*. Toronto: Inner City Books, 1985.

The Life Course and Life Transitions

Becker, Gay. *Growing Old in Silence*. Berkeley, CA: University of California Press, 1980.

Brim, Orville and S. Wheeler. *Socialization After Childhood*. New York: Wiley, 1966.

Clark, M. Margaret and Barbara G. Anderson. *Culture and Aging*. Springfield, IL: Charles C. Thomas, 1967.

Erikson, Erik H. *Childhood and Society*. New York: W. W. Norton, 1950.

George, Linda K. "Models of Transitions in Middle and Later Life." *The Annals of the American Academy of Political and Social Science*, 464:22–37, 1982.

Hultsch, David F. and Judy K. Plemons. "Life Events and

Life-Span Development." In Paul B. Baltes and Orville Brim, Jr., eds., *Life-Span Development and Behavior*. Volume 2. New York: Academic Press, 1979, pp. 1–36.

Kaufman, Sharon R. *The Ageless Self*. Madison, WI: University of Wisconsin Press, 1987.

Levinson, Daniel J., C. M. Darrow, E. B. Klein, M. H. Levinson, and B. McKee. *Seasons of a Man's Life*. New York: Knopf, 1978.

Marris, Peter. *Loss and Change*. London: Routledge & Kegan Paul, 1974.

Neugarten, Bernice. "Adaptation and the Life Cycle." *The Counseling Psychologist*, 6, No. 1, 1976.

———. "The Awareness of Middle Age." In Bernice Neugarten, ed., *Middle Age and Aging*. Chicago: University of Chicago Press, 1968, pp. 93–98.

———. "Time, Age, and the Life Cycle." *American Journal of Psychiatry*, 136:887–893, 1979.

Parkes, C. Murray. "Psycho-social Transitions: A Field for Study." *Social Science and Medicine*, 5:101–105, 1971.

Pearlin, Leonard I. "Discontinuities in the Study of Aging." In Tamara Hareven and Kathleen J. Adams, eds., *Aging and Life Course Transitions: An Interdisciplinary Perspective*. New York: Guilford Press, 1982, pp. 55–74.

General

Becker, Gay and Regina Arnold. "Stigma as a Social and Cultural Construct." In Stephen Ainlay, Gay Becker, and Lerita Coleman, eds., *The Dilemma of Difference: A Multidisciplinary View of Stigma*. New York: Plenum Press, 1985, pp. 37–59.

Geertz, Clifford. *The Interpretation of Cultures*. New York: Basic Books, 1973.

Goffman, Erving. *Stigma: Notes on the Management of Spoiled Identity*. Englewood Cliffs, NJ: Prentice-Hall, 1963.

Hallowell, A. Irving. *Culture and Experience*. Philadelphia: University of Pennsylvania Press, 1955.

Spradley, James P. and David W. McCurdy. *Conformity and Conflict: Readings in Cultural Anthropology*. Boston, MA: Little, Brown, 1971.

Websters' New World Dictionary of the American Language. New York: Simon & Schuster, 1982.

INDEX

www.ingramcontent.com/pod-product-compliance
Lightning Source LLC
LaVergne TN
LVHW100251210926
848480LV00003B/898
* 9 7 8 0 5 2 0 3 3 5 3 8 7 *